Etiology, Prevention and Management of Cardiomyopathy

Edited by Ernest A. Adeghate

Published in London, United Kingdom

Etiology, Prevention and Management of Cardiomyopathy
http://dx.doi.org/10.5772/intechopen.1001769
Edited by Ernest A. Adeghate

Contributors
Abla Ismail, Ahmed Bin Amar, Aishwarya Singh, Alexandru Mihai Cornea, Alina Ligia Cornea, Carlin Hanoman, Chris Sawh, Cristian Daniel Rodríguez, Cristian Orlando Porras Bueno, Emanuel Cummings, Ernest A. Adeghate, Ernst von Schwarz, Guillermo Belerenian, Guillermo Rodriguez, Gustavo Abuin, Hazel Contractor, Jaipaul Singh, Kamaldeep Singh, Khemraj Rupee, Mabel Lucero Olarte Jurado, Manal Smail, Mariam AlOtaiba, Monika Moni, Mustafa Kaplangoray, Omobola Awosika Oyeleye, Raphael Singh, Rohit Mishra, Sahar Mohsin, Suhail AlAmry, Sunil Rupee, Víctor Castillo

First published in London, United Kingdom, 2024 by IntechOpen
IntechOpen is the global imprint of INTECHOPEN LIMITED, registered in England and Wales, registration number: 11086078, 167-169 Great Portland Street, London, W1W 5PF, United Kingdom

British Library Cataloguing-in-Publication Data
A catalogue record for this book is available from the British Library

Additional hard and PDF copies can be obtained from orders@intechopen.com

Etiology, Prevention and Management of Cardiomyopathy
Edited by Ernest A. Adeghate
p. cm.

This title is part of the Cardiology and Cardiovascular Medicine Book Series, Volume 6
Topic: Cardiovascular Diseases and Health
Series Editor: Kaan Kırali
Topic Editor: Mahi L. Ashwath

Print ISBN 978-0-85466-911-0
Online ISBN 978-0-85466-910-3
eBook (PDF) ISBN 978-0-85466-912-7
ISSN 3033-361X

For EU product safety concerns:
IN TECH d.o.o., Prolaz Marije Krucifikse Kozulić 3, 51000 Rijeka, Croatia,
info@intechopen.com or visit our website at intechopen.com.

IntechOpen Book Series

Cardiology and Cardiovascular Medicine

Volume 6

Aims and Scope of the Series

Today, since molecular science on structural causes of oncological pathologies and their molecular treatments are developing at an unbelievable rate, the primary medical cause of death in the twenty-first century will be cardiovascular disease. Neither pandemics that threaten all humanity nor deterioration in the ecosystem will be able to change this fact. Especially, this century seems poised to witness an incredible struggle against atherosclerotic disease, which develops in the arterial walls and results in narrowing and occlusion of the arterial lumen. In addition to this disease, there has been an increasing prevalence of heart rhythm problems, deterioration of heart valves due to aging, and heart failure. Serious vascular pathologies such as stenosis and occlusion, dissection and rupture, and aneurysmal enlargement are also major concerns. Medical and invasive treatment methods may work to save human lives, but they will never provide a real solution. All kinds of medical, technological, and genetic engineering developments obtained in these processes have not yet been sufficient to alleviate or eliminate cardiovascular disease. This book series, Cardiology and Cardiovascular Medicine, includes three topics. The first, Cardiovascular Diseases and Health, reviews important cardiovascular diseases and the developments in their prognosis. The second topic, Cardiovascular Electrophysiology, illuminates the abnormal functioning of the cardiac conduction system, which is caused by all heart pathologies and negatively affects prognosis. The third topic in this series, Cardiovascular Surgery, details treatment for cardiovascular pathologies and how to regulate normal physiological functions with percutaneous or extracorporeal interventions.

Meet the Series Editor

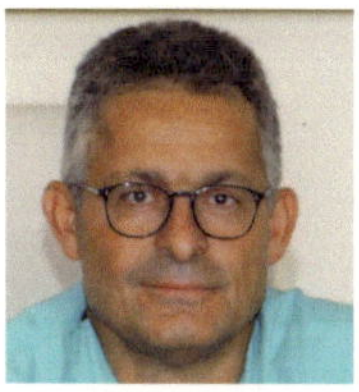

After completing his studies at the Medicine Faculty of Istanbul University in 1990, Prof. Kaan Kırali fulfilled his mandatory medical service and commenced his residency training at Koşuyolu Heart and Research Hospital in 1992. Following five years of assistant education, he pursued further training in England and the USA in 1998. Specializing in laparoscopic and minimally invasive cardiac surgery, he earned the titles of consultant cardiovascular surgeon in 1998, Assistant Professor in 1999, Associate Professor in 2002, and Chief in 2005 at the same hospital. Prof. Kırali also developed an interest in preventive medicine, obtaining an MSc in Public Health from Istanbul University in 2000. Over the past two decades, he has concentrated his scientific pursuits on cardiovascular repairs requiring specialized experience. With his expertise in coronary artery surgery, minimally invasive cardiac surgery, valve repair, and aortic root surgery, he has established new methods for awake coronary bypass revascularization, a new surgical approach for AVR during first and re-operations, aortic valve-sparing procedure, and radiofrequency ablation. Notably, he pioneered awake complete coronary artery bypass grafting (CABG) with bilateral internal mammary arteries (BIMA) and played a crucial role in advancing aortic root surgery with a new aortotomy incision, simplifying aortic valve interventions. Since the year 2000, Prof. Kırali has expanded his interests to heart transplantation, and in recent years, to left ventricular assist devices. He has served as the head of the transplantation department since 2015 and currently continues his work as the director of Koşuyolu High Specialization Education and Research Hospital in Istanbul, Turkey. In his prolific career, he has authored numerous papers in SCI journals, contributed to various book chapters, and served as an editor and reviewer for multiple academic journals. Additionally, he has edited several international books in the field of cardiovascular medicine.

Meet the Volume Editor

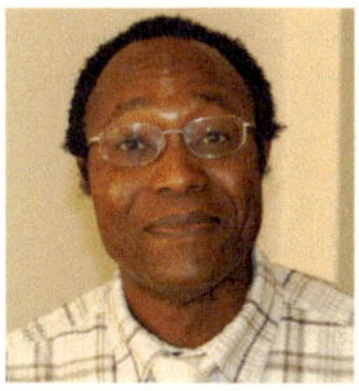

Dr. Adeghate obtained his MD from Semmelweis University Medical School, Budapest, Hungary and his Ph.D. and DSc from the Hungarian Academy of Sciences. He has a master of family medicine degree from Monash University, Australia. Dr. Adeghate is a professor at the College of Medicine & Health Sciences, United Arab Emirates University, Al Ain, United Arab Emirates, and a past chairperson of the Diabetes and Cardiovascular Research Priority Group, United Arab Emirates University. His research interest is in the field of experimental diabetes, and he has published more than 250 full-length articles in peer-reviewed journals as well as 15 book chapters. He edited a book entitled Diabetes Mellitus & Its Complications: Molecular Mechanisms, Epidemiology & Clinical Medicine, which was published in 2006.

Contents

Preface

Cardiomyopathy (CM) is a common condition affecting millions of people worldwide. It was reported that one in every 500 people suffers from dilated or hypertrophic cardiomyopathy. CM occurs when either the structure or the function of cardiomyocytes is impaired. The causes of CM are diverse and could include infection (viral, fungal, or bacterial), genetic mutations of the building blocks (actin, myosin) of cardiomyocytes, and remodeling of the extracellular matrix of the myocardium. In addition, myocarditis has been classified as a type of cardiomyopathy because of the ability of condition to cause scars or damage the myocardium to the extent that will make it impossible to perform its function. Conditions such as amyloidosis, sarcoidosis, and hemochromatosis can also induced cardiomyopathy by their ability to form granulomas, nodules, and space-occupying lesions in the myocardial layer of the heart. The weaking of heart muscles as seen in the case of muscular dystrophy can also lead to cardiomyopathy that grossly impairs the function of the heart. Any condition such as abnormally high lipid levels in the blood can cause coronary artery disease leading to cardiomyopathy.

The onset of cardiomyopathy leads to a different array of signs and symptoms that grossly affect the well-being and the standard of living of the patient, depending on the severity of the condition. These symptoms include but are not limited to arrhythmias, chest pain, difficult breathing, and ankle edema. If severe, these symptoms may culminate in heart failure and eventually sudden cardiac death. It is worth noting that cardiac diseases including cardiomyopathy are the most common cause of death globally.

The first chapter, "Cardiomyopathies: A Historical Journey", presents a broad overview of cardiomyopathy. The chapter discusses how experts in the field of cardiology arrived at the classification of cardiomyopathy that continues to evolve to this day. The chapter also analyzed how the European Society of Cardiology and the American Heart Association arrived at the current classification of cardiomyopathy. The authors of this chapter concluded that the classification of cardiomyopathy is based on a structural–functional premise, which is important to the management of cardiomyopathy. The second chapter is entitled, "Cardiomyopathy: Exploring the Causes, Prevention and Management of Cardiomyopathy". The authors of this chapter list different types of cardiomyopathies, including dilated, hypertrophic, restrictive, arrhythmogenic, and lastly Takotsubo cardiomyopathy. They also present the causes, diagnosis, clinical presentations, and management of each of these types of cardiomyopathies. Of note is the use of SGLT2 inhibitors to improve cardiac function irrespective of the presence of diabetes mellitus. The use of beta and calcium channel blockers is recommended for the treatment of most cardiomyopathies.

Chapter 3, entitled "Understanding Cardiomyopathy: Epidemiology, Risk Factors, Types, Mechanisms, Diagnosis, Prevention, and Treatment", was written by Jaipaul Singh et al. The authors identify key lifestyle modifications that can help alleviate the signs and symptoms of cardiomyopathy. These include dietary changes, reduced alcohol intake, abstinence from tobacco use, reduced stress intensity, healthy weight, psychological interventions, and consistent physical activity. The authors conclude that angiotensin-converting enzyme inhibitors and loop diuretics are commonly used to treat patients suffering from cardiomyopathy.

Chapter 4 of this book is “Cardiomyopathy with Subclinical Heart Failure”. The chapter explores both primary and secondary cardiomyopathies and how these could lead to heart failure. In addition, the chapter gave a detailed description of pharmacological and surgical regimens available for the treatment of cardiomyopathies.

Chapter 5, “Diabetes-Induced Cardiomyopathy: Updates in Epidemiology, Prevention and Management”. examines how diabetic cardiomyopathy could be held back with healthy diet, physical exercise, sleep, reduction of stress, and abstinence from smoking and alcohol. The authors concluded that GLP-1 receptor agonists with or without SGLT2 inhibitors are useful in the treatment of diabetic cardiomyopathy. Chapter 6, entitled “Left Ventricle Arrhythmogenic Cardiomyopathy in Canines and Felines” proves that the signs and symptoms of cardiomyopathy observed in humans are also present in companion animals. Chapter 7, “Premature Ventricular Complex-Induced/-Aggravated Cardiomyopathy”, delves into the etiology, diagnosis, clinical presentations, and management of premature ventricular complex-induced/aggravated cardiomyopathy.

Chapter 8, entitled “Comprehensive Interventions in End-Stage Cardiomyopathy: Mechanical Circulatory Support and Heart Transplantation”, analyzes the indications, methods, and rationale for using mechanical support and heart transplantation to treat patients with end-stage cardiomyopathy.

I sincerely thank all contributing authors. I would like to take this opportunity to express my profound gratitude to Ms. Ivana Barac, the publishing process manager, for processing and preparation of this book. My thank also goes to Ms. Jelena Germuth in facilitating the initiation of the book.

Ernest A. Adeghate MD, Ph.D.
College of Medicine and Health Sciences,
United Arab Emirates University,
Al Ain, United Arab Emirates

Chapter 1

Cardiomyopathies: A Historical Journey

Cristian Orlando Porras Bueno and Mabel Lucero Olarte Jurado

Abstract

This chapter in question provides a comprehensive overview of the evolution of cardiomyopathy classifications, tracing the historical development of key concepts that have shaped the primary categorizations recognized in medical literature. It offers a critical analysis of the present state of cardiomyopathy classifications, exploring the nuances and contentious points within the latest frameworks proposed by leading health authorities such as the European Society of Cardiology (ESC) and the American Heart Association (AHA). The narrative also encompasses the inception and transformation of the term 'cardiomyopathy' itself, culminating in the adoption of morphological-functional types that are crucial to the clinical management of these heart muscle disorders.

Keywords: cardiomyopathies, history, books, classification, cardiomyopathy hypertrophic, cardiomyopathy dilated, cardiomyopathy restrictive, arrhythmogenic right ventricular dysplasia

Methodology

We perform a review of the available medical literature in the major clinical databases PubMed, Google Scholar, and SciELO, using the mesh terms "cardiomyopathies," "history," and "classification" in PubMed and Google Scholar and the analogous Spanish terms of "cardiomyopathies" and "classification" in SciELO. We found 239 articles in PubMed, 50 articles in the first five pages of Google Scholar and 3 articles in SciELO, which contained the previously mesh terms. After being read one by one by each of the authors, 24 articles were selected that included in their content information related to the history of cardiomyopathies and their classification schemes.

1. Introduction

The importance of understanding the historical evolution of cardiomyopathies, a group of diseases that affect the heart muscle, has been a subject of medical research and discussion for many years [1]. The historical evolution of cardiomyopathies is a critical area of study within cardiovascular medicine, reflecting a journey of discovery that has significantly enhanced our understanding of heart diseases [2].

Initially, cardiomyopathies were primarily recognized as distinct diseases of the heart muscle, not attributable to the common causes of heart dysfunction such as hypertension, valvular, or congenital heart disease. Over time, the definition has expanded and now includes a diverse group of conditions characterized by their genetic, structural, and functional heterogeneity [2].

The term "cardiomyopathy" was first used in 1957 [3] by Wallace Bridgen, marking the beginning of a more detailed categorization and understanding of heart muscle diseases. A few years later, in 1968, cardiomyopathies were described as "diseases of different and often unknown aetiology in which the dominant feature was cardiomegaly and heart failure" by the World Health Organization (WHO) [4].

Over the years, the classification of cardiomyopathies has evolved significantly. The original 1980 WHO classification defined cardiomyopathies as "heart muscle diseases of unknown cause," reflecting the limited knowledge of the time [5]. This definition has since expanded, and the classification has become more nuanced, incorporating genetic, mixed, and acquired categories, as well as recognizing cardiomyopathies as part of systemic diseases.

Then, in 2006, the American Heart Association (AHA) classification was considered as the gold standard for several years. It was developed in response to the explosion of knowledge in the field, particularly with the advent of modern molecular biology, which has provided a deeper understanding of the genetic and phenotypic expressions of these diseases. This classification system has been instrumental in guiding research and treatment, offering a framework for understanding the complex and heterogeneous nature of cardiomyopathies [6]. Furthermore, 2 years later, the 2008 European Society of Cardiology (ESC) classification was published in response to the statements described above [7].

Finally, it is important to highlight the recently developed 2023 cardiomyopathies ESC guidelines because a new classification of these diseases was developed, taking into account new emerging evidence, which allowed us to introduce new emerging concepts such as the nondilated left ventricular cardiomyopathy classification, the exclusion of left ventricular noncompacted cardiomyopathy from the main classification, and also the change in the way to refer to takotsubo syndrome, among others [8].

The previously described advances underline the importance of the historical evolution of cardiomyopathy classifications over time, as a paradigm shift has occurred from a one-size-fits-all clinical approach to a more precise phenotypic and genotypic classification, with a detailed description focused on the morphological and functional characteristics of the myocardium, which has allowed a comprehensive approach and diagnosis, as well as individualized treatment, based on the most up-to-date information.

Likewise, it is essential to recognize that, with the advancement of research, the historical perspective will likely maintain its value, guiding future classifications, hand in hand with the advent of evidence derived from the development of new technologies in this field of study. Below, we describe a more detailed perspective on the past, present, and future of cardiomyopathies.

2. Cardiomyopathies: a retrospective review

Although the name cardiomyopathy was first used in 1957 by Wallace Bridgen to refer to non-coronary myocardial diseases of uncertain etiology [3], it should be noted that prior to this, at the end of the 19th century, the term chronic myocarditis was used to refer to any disease of the heart muscle of non-valvular origin as the only recognized myocardial pathology [4]. Later, in Germany in 1891, Krehl coined the concept of idiopathic diseases of the cardiac muscle, and in 1901, in Lyon, France, Josseran and Gallavardin introduced the term primary myocardial disease when myocardial involvement of idiopathic etiology occurred [4].

Years later, in 1933, Warren noted the peculiarity of the diagnosis confirmation of chronic myocarditis in autopsies, prompting research attention to non-inflammatory pathologies, particularly arterial hypertension and coronary heart disease. Warren also warned of two causes of death in cardiomyopathies: sudden death or progressive deterioration of cardiorespiratory failure [9]. H. Christian pointed out later in 1950 that a third of non-inflammatory heart illnesses were not attributable to arterial hypertension or coronary heart disease, which is why this category of disorders with unclear causes came to be known as primary myocardial disease [10, 11].

It should be noted that in 1956, Blankenhorn and Gall used the term myocarditis to refer to the inflammatory pathology of the cardiac muscle and myocardosis to the cardiac pathologies of degenerative etiology [12]. It is at this historical moment that, for the first time in 1957, Wallace Bridgen used the term cardiomyopathy, as previously mentioned [3]. Wallace used the term to refer to non-coronary myocardial illness, dividing it into five categories based on the source: congenital, infectious, caused by amyloidosis, collagen disease, and an anatomical variety of endomyocardial fibrosis of idiopathic etiology.

Moreover, he was adamant about limiting the term "myocarditis" to infectious myocardial pathologies and predicted that the category of "idiopathic cardiomyopathies" would gradually diminish as different causative agents were identified [3]. Afterward, in 1961, J.F. Goodwin et al. defined myocardiopathies as sub-acute or chronic diseases of the cardiac muscle with unknown etiology. Also, for the first time, they classified the cardiomyopathies into three forms: Congestive, which will be recognized currently as dilated cardiomyopathy; obliterated or constrictive, which is currently recognized as restrictive cardiomyopathy; and obstructive, which is recognized today as hypertrophic cardiomyopathy [13].

Subsequently, the WHO began using the term "cardiomyopathy" in 1968 to refer to myocardial disease with an unclear etiology that was characterized by cardiomegaly and heart failure [14]. In 1972, Oakley and Goodwin defined cardiomyopathy as a heart muscle disorder of unknown cause [15], also classifying it into three groups, as was previously realized by Goodwin in 1961 [13]. Moreover, this classification was the first to propose a treatment based on one of these three classifications (congestive cardiomyopathy, hypertrophic cardiomyopathy, and obliterative).

However, it is crucial to note that, prior to the uniform use of the term hypertrophic cardiomyopathy, no fewer than 58 names or terms were used to refer to hypertrophic cardiomyopathy [16], which denoted, for that date, the need to continue evolving in the unification of terminology and the proposal of classifications for these pathologies.

Regarding the treatment of congestive cardiomyopathy, Oakley and Goodwin proposed in 1972 that the mainstays were bed rest, digitals, and diuretics [13]. With respect to the treatment of hypertrophic cardiomyopathy, they proposed a surgical approach with an incision or excision of the hypertrophied septum when left ventricular outflow tract obstruction was present; however, this approach only demonstrated improvement in symptoms to date; they also proposed beta blockers for the treatment of angina [13].

Due to the limited understanding of cardiac diseases at the time, the WHO/International Society and Federation of Cardiology (ISFC) Task Force defined cardiomyopathy as heart muscle diseases of unknown etiology in 1980 and proposed a new classification system for the condition [5]; In it, cardiomyopathies were classified as dilated, hypertrophic, and restrictive, also highlighting that these three categories should be differentiated from unclassified cardiomyopathy.

The term unclassified cardiomyopathy comprises certain heart muscle illnesses with a recognized cause or linked to systemic diseases, as well as latent cardiomyopathy with early cardiac abnormalities. Besides, systemic and pulmonary hypertension, as well as coronary artery disease (CAD), valvulopathies, and congenital cardiac diseases, were excluded from this classification [5]. This classification is illustrated in **Figure 1**.

Nevertheless, some years later, a revised categorization of cardiac disorders was released by the WHO/ISFC Task Force in 1996, taking account of the new knowledge about the pathophysiology, etiology, and/or pathogenesis of these conditions. It described cardiomyopathy as a myocardial disease linked to cardiac dysfunction and classified cardiomyopathies into four distinct categories: restricted, dilated, and hypertrophic cardiomyopathy, and also included the first description of arrhythmogenic right ventricular cardiomyopathy [17].

Also, among other unclassified cardiomyopathies that did not fall into these four previously described categories, noncompacted myocardium, mitochondrial

WHO/ISFC Classification 1980

Tipe of cardiomyopathy*	Mechanical dysfunction	Left ventricular volume	Ejection fraction	Parietal thickness
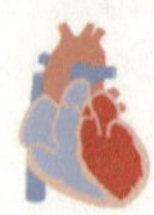 Dilated	Systolic	Increased	20-40%	Normal or decreased
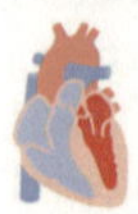 Hypertrophic	Diastolic	Decreased or markedly increased	57-70%	Markedly increased
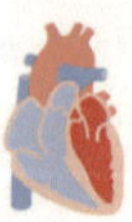 Restrictive	Diastolic	Normal or decreased	50-60%	Normal or increased

Figure 1.
*1980 WHO/ISFC classification of the three main types of cardiomyopathies and their main characteristics. *The three main categories of this classification are described; however, unclassified and specific disease categories are also included. WHO = World Health Organization. ISFC = International Society and Federation of Cardiology.*

fibroelastosis, and systolic dysfunction with mild dilatation were included [17]. Furthermore, this classification included specific cardiomyopathies, previously known as particular heart muscle diseases, which are associated with specific conditions or systemic disorders. Moreover, there was confusion regarding the classification of cardiac disorders because ischaemic, valvular, and hypertensive cardiomyopathies were grouped together under the heading of specific cardiomyopathies.

3. Cardiomyopathies: a current vision

Currently, in the 21st century, several classifications have been developed, highlighting among them the 2006 AHA classification [6], the 2008 ESC classification [7], the classification proposed in 2013 by Arbustini et al. [18, 19], and the recently published classification in 2023 by the ESC [8] which are described below. The strengths and weaknesses of the currently mainly used classifications are presented in **Table 1**.

In 2006, the AHA released a scientific statement that included a new categorization for cardiomyopathies based on advancements in genetic testing and diagnostic imaging techniques in cardiology [6]. This scientific statement was developed to improve communication between researchers and clinicians while also describing novel cardiac diseases, including conduction system disorders and channelopathies, which were described for the first time.

According to the 2006 AHA consensus, cardiomyopathies are a heterogeneous group of cardiac disorders that are often inherited and linked to mechanical or electrical dysfunction, considering that they can either be systemic or limited to the heart [6].

Also, each cardiomyopathy category was divided into two subcategories (primary or secondary) according to whether it was inherited, acquired, or secondary to a systemic disease: A primary cardiomyopathy refers to a confined heart disease and is divided into genetic, mixed (genetic and nongenetic), and acquired. Regarding secondary cardiomyopathies, they were described as part of systemic diseases that were previously referred to as "specific cardiomyopathies" [6]. The current AHA classification for primary cardiomyopathies is illustrated in **Figure 2**.

Two years later, in 2008, the ESC published a new classification that included a revised definition for cardiomyopathy: a cardiac disease marked by an abnormal myocardium both structurally and functionally. The five clinically oriented phenotypes that comprise this new categorization of cardiomyopathies are restricted, hypertrophic, dilated, arrhythmogenic right ventricular cardiomyopathy (ARVC), and unclassified [7].

Additionally, the new ESC consensus classified myocardiopathies as either nonfamilial or familial, with familial defined as occurring in several family members or exhibiting a phenotype that may be due to the same genetic mutation. It is important to highlight that the initial occurrence of a mutation is what defines sporadic genetic cardiomyopathy. Nonfamilial cardiomyopathy, which can be classified as either idiopathic or acquired, is defined by the absence of associated family history [7]. Furthermore, it is also critical to recognize that the difference between cardiomyopathies and specific heart muscle diseases was abandoned at this historical moment.

Furthermore, it is important to note that the 2006 AHA classification may make it difficult to distinguish between primary and secondary cardiomyopathies and understand the causes of cardiac diseases. This is because systemic symptoms can occur in primary cardiomyopathies and vice versa, and channelopathies may not produce morphofunctional phenotypes and thus should not be classified as distinct cardiomyopathies.

Classification	Strengths	Weaknesses
AHA 2006	• Adopts the division into primary cardiomyopathies and secondary cardiomyopathies with a clinical context criterion. • Systemic diseases associated with secondary forms of cardiomyopathies, previously referred to as "specific cardiomyopathies," have been excluded from this classification.	• Weak SCD risk assessment. • These guidelines do not include recommendations for exercise or pregnancy. • Inclusion of other traits and syndromes as cardiomyopathies, which to date are not considered cardiomyopathies by other scientific associations, for example, myocarditis, LVNC, and takotsubo syndrome.
MOGE(S) 2013	• Assessment of morphofunctional type, systems involved, genetic or familial inheritance pattern, etiology, and functional status.	• Non-inclusion of tachycardiomyopathy, cardiomyopathy associated with endocrine diseases, and peripartum cardiomyopathy in its etiological classification. • Neither assessment of phenotypes nor severity of ventricular dysfunction. • Weak SCD risk assessment.
ESC 2023	• Phenotypic approach to cardiomyopathies based on morphological and functional characteristics of the myocardium. • Improvements in imaging methods, supporting CMR at diagnosis in all cases with a level IB recommendation, and taking into account repeating it every 2–5 years. • Highlights of the key role of ventricular myocardial scar assessment using CMR. • It is emphasized the significance of genetic testing because it can be used for diagnosis, prognosis, and treatment of several cardiomyopathies. • New recommendations on SCD risk stratification for different cardiomyopathy phenotypes, also highlighting the important role of genotype in the SCD risk assessment. • Exercise and pregnancy recommendations are included in the guidelines. • New emerging concepts: NDLVC as a new cardiomyopathy phenotype; LVNC excluded as cardiomyopathy and considered a ventricular phenotype; and stress cardiomyopathy or Takotsubo syndrome is not recommended to be classified as a cardiomyopathy.	• The novel concept of NDLVC presents difficulties with regard to treatment recommendations and arrhythmic stratification due to its genetic and mechanistic heterogeneity. Furthermore, the fact that CMR is needed for diagnosis makes calculating its prevalence difficult. • Despite the CMR recommendation at diagnosis in all cases, it is not widely available for all patients. Also, there are still gaps with CMR, such as the future impact of it on screening and how to standardize LGE quantification.

AHA = American Heart Association. CMR = Cardiac magnetic resonance. ESC = European Society of Cardiology. LGE = Late gadolinium enhancement. LVNC = Left ventricular non-compaction. NDLVC = Nondilated left ventricular cardiomyopathy. SCD = Sudden cardiac death.

Table 1.
Strengths and weaknesses of current cardiomyopathies classifications.

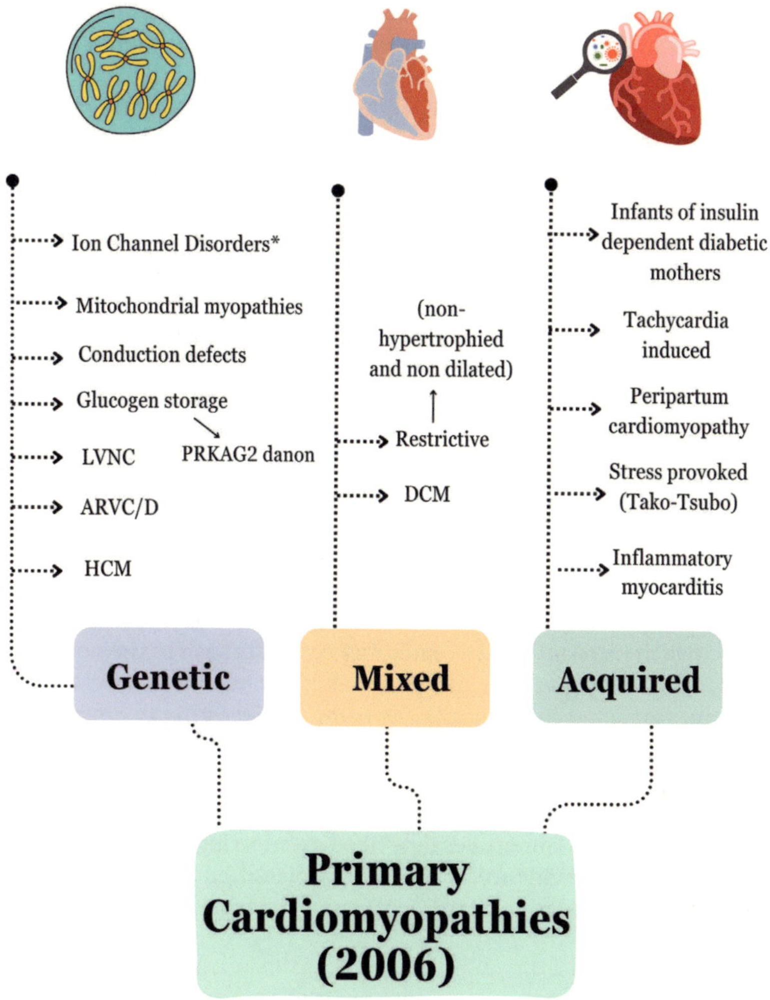

Figure 2.
*2006 AHA proposed classification for primary cardiomyopathies. *Ion Channel Disorders include long QT syndrome, short QT syndrome, Brugada syndrome, Catecholaminergic Polymorphic Ventricular Tachycardia and Asian sudden unexplained nocturnal death syndrome. AHA = American Heart Association.*

Moreover, though there are many similarities between the two systems and significant recommendations, the 2006 AHA categorization scheme describes cardiomyopathies by first describing the underlying genetics of the etiology and then going on to detail the phenotypic aspects of cardiac involvement [6]. On the other hand, the 2008 ESC categorization scheme has kept its basic morphofunctional categories and further divided them into nongenetic (nonfamilial) and genetic (familial) divisions [7].

Furthermore, in 2013, Arbustini et al. proposed a new classification scheme denominated MOGE (S), which resembles the TNM staging system used for cancer. M stands for morphofunctional type, O for organ or system involvement, G for genetic or familial inheritance pattern, and E for etiology and functional status (S) [18, 19]. The proposed scheme uses the New York Heart Association functional classes (I–IV) and the American College of Cardiology (ACC)/AHA (A-D), respectively, for the functional status. Cardiomyopathy, according to Arbustini et al., is characterized by an abnormal myocardium in both morphology and function when no other diseases are present, which leads to this.

Despite the main advantage of the MOGE(S) proposed scheme [18, 19], which allows a global evaluation of cardiomyopathy, this new scheme has several limitations: One of these is the non-inclusion of tachycardiomyopathy, cardiomyopathy associated with endocrine diseases, and peripartum cardiomyopathy in its etiological classification. In addition, the dynamic assessment of phenotypes and the early phases of myocardial disease are not embraced. Lastly, it does not address the severity of ventricular dysfunction, which may affect the course of treatment and prognosis for these patients, acute heart failure, or the risk of sudden death, which is common in cardiomyopathies. Possibly due to the several limitations described above, the MOGE(S) classification has not been widely used by clinicians and researchers across the world.

Along with genetic development, genetics research has made significant achievements in 2016, defining the molecular origins of cardiomyopathies [20]. For hypertrophic, dilated, restricted, and arrhythmogenic cardiomyopathies, more than a 1000 mutations in numerous genes with different ontologies have been found. These mutations allowed us to discover the various molecules and pathways involved in the development of cardiomyopathies [20].

Finally, last year, the ESC released its last cardiomyopathies guideline with its classification, which introduced new emerging concepts such as the nondilated left ventricular cardiomyopathy in the main classification and the exclusion of the left ventricular noncompacted cardiomyopathy from it, suggesting to refer to it as left ventricular hypertrabeculation because, with emerging evidence, it is currently considered a phenotype in itself rather than a cardiomyopathy [8].

As well, this new guideline recommends abolishing the use of the term "stress cardiomyopathy," which is sometimes described as referring to Tako-tsubo syndrome, which, in light of current evidence, should not be classified as a cardiomyopathy. The current ESC classification for myocardiopathies is illustrated in **Figure 3**.

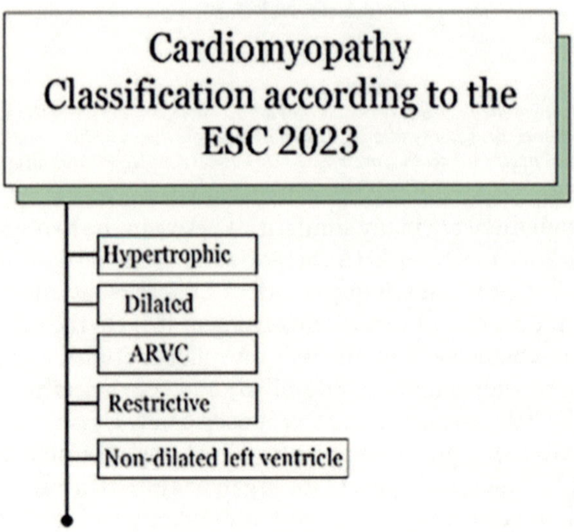

Figure 3.
Cardiomyopathies classification according to the 2023 ESC guidelines. ARVC = Arrhythmogenic right ventricular cardiomyopathy. ESC = European Society of Cardiology.

Furthermore, even though there have been significant advancements in cardiomyopathy diagnosis, treatment, and genetics in the past several years, there are still a number of areas where strong evidence is still lacking and should be the focus of future clinical research [8].

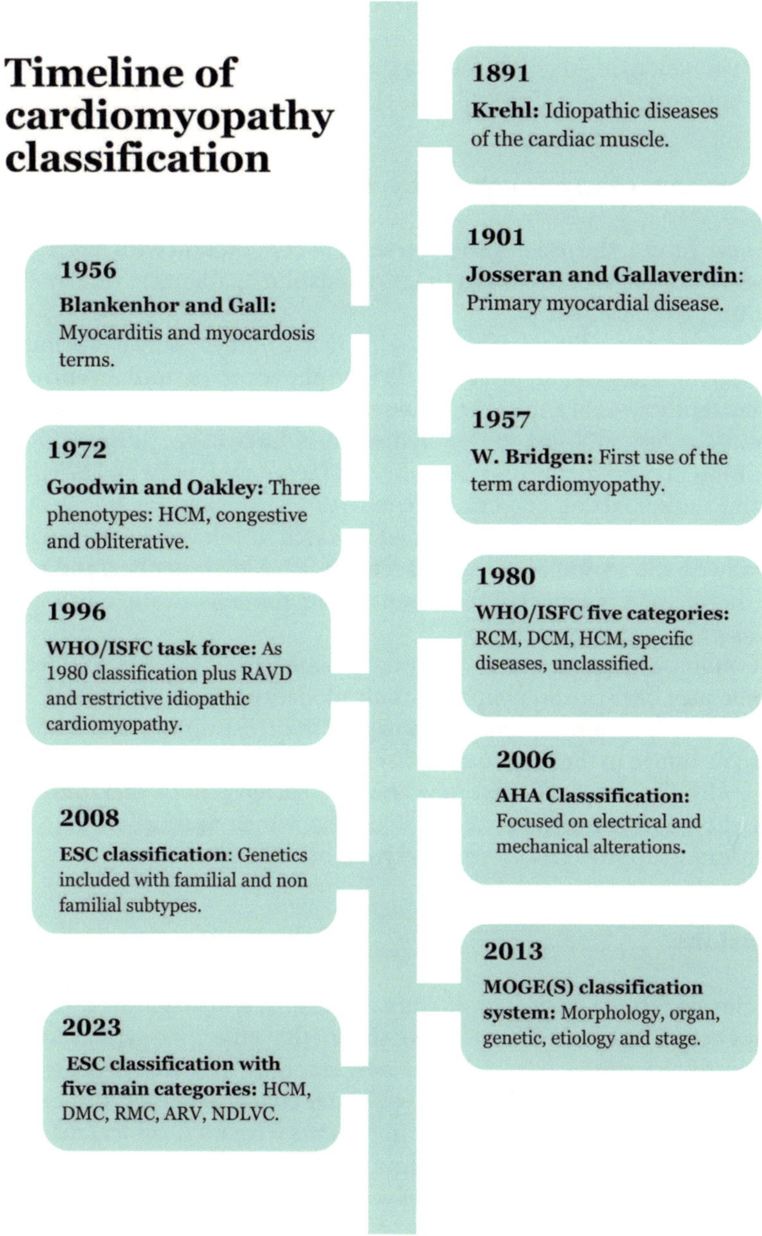

Figure 4.
Timeline of cardiomyopathy classification. HCM = Hypertrophic cardiomyopathy. DMC = Dilated cardiomyopathy. RMC = Restrictive cardiomyopathy. ARV = Arrhythmogenic right ventricular cardiomyopathy. ESC = European Society of Cardiology. NDLVC = Nondilated left ventricular cardiomyopathy. WHO = World Health Organization. ISFC = International Society and Federation of Cardiology.

Likewise, it is important to highlight that although these ESC guidelines have had general global acceptance, some scientific societies, such as the Spanish Society of Cardiology, have made comments regarding what the consequences of implementing them in Spain would be, mainly describing limitations with the use of CMR, the quantification of late gadolinium enhancement (LGE), and the availability of genetic tests, among others [21]. Therefore, it is important to analyze and apply each contextualized and individualized recommendation to each patient, as well as to the resources available in each centre.

Finally, we want to highlight, through a timeline, the conceptual evolution that the term cardiomyopathy has had, as well as its classification which is illustrated in **Figure 4**.

4. Classifications of cardiomyopathy: their future directions

In the near future, the use of genetic testing in conjunction with hybrid cardiac imaging will be important in clinical practice, enabling patients to receive therapy, diagnosis, and prognosis early.

Regarding genetics, clinical genetic testing in cardiomyopathy has primarily been used to screen families and identify rare disease phenocopies until recently. However, there are currently several clinical trials assessing gene therapy for cardiomyopathies such those secondary to X-linked Danon disease, X-linked Fabry disease, X-linked Duchenne muscular dystrophy disease, autosomal recessive Pompe and Friedreich ataxia diseases, and autosomal dominant transthyretin (TTR) amyloidosis among others [22].

In conjunction with the aforementioned research, it is factually reasonable to believe that with the advent of gene replacement, RNA therapeutics, and novel small-molecule therapies, it is expected that determining the genetic etiology will play a key role in managing cardiomyopathies [22].

Furthermore, when it comes to the initial assessment, diagnosis, and treatment of patients who may have cardiomyopathy, multimodality imaging is crucial. Because of this, the development of multimodality imaging in care, training, and research will be essential to its future in the diagnosis and treatment of cardiomyopathies [23].

Finally, with the advent of these new etiology-driven genetic therapies and imaging approaches, new emerging concepts will arise, which could allow us to propose new classification approaches for cardiomyopathies in a few years.

5. Conclusions

In conclusion, after a critical evaluation of the different classifications of cardiomyopathies proposed, these schemes have shown that emerging gaps are a constant across this cardiology topic. However, the new emerging research in genetic and imaging aspects, among others, will allow a better characterization and understanding of these complex diseases, especially in patients with mild clinical manifestations, early stages, dynamic presentation, or those with mixed phenotypes.

Acknowledgements

To the Autonomous University of Bucaramanga (UNAB) and the Pontifical Xavierian University (PUJ) for promoting publication and research. Besides, this chapter book has been funded by the authors.

Conflict of interest

The authors declare no conflict of interest.

Author details

Cristian Orlando Porras Bueno[1*] and Mabel Lucero Olarte Jurado[2]

1 Pontifical Xavierian University (PUJ), Bogotá, Colombia

2 Autonomous University of Bucaramanga (UNAB), Floridablanca, Colombia

*Address all correspondence to: cporras186@unab.edu.co

References

[1] Maron BJ. Is the 2006 American Heart Association classification of cardiomyopathies the gold standard? Circulatory Failure. 2008;**1**(1):72-76

[2] Cury Salemi VM, Mohty D, Lustosa de Altavila SL, Tavares de Melo MD, Kalil Filho R, Bocchi EA. Insights into the classification of cardiomyopathies: Past, present, and future directions. Clinics. 2021;**76**:e2808

[3] Brigden W. Uncommon myocardial diseases: The non-coronary cardiomyopathies. Lancet. 1957;**273**(7008):1243-1249

[4] Abelmann WH. Classification and natural history of primary myocardial disease. Progress in Cardiovascular Diseases. 1984;**27**(2):73-94

[5] Bradenburg R, Chazov E, Cherian G, Falase A, Grosgogeat Y, Kawai C, et al. Report of the WHO/ISFC task force on the definition and classification of cardiomyopathies. British Heart Journal. 1980;**44**(6):672-673

[6] Maron BJ, Towbin JA, Thiene G, Antzelevitch C, Corrado D, Arnett D, et al. Contemporary definitions and classification of the cardiomyopathies: An American Heart Association scientific statement from the council on clinical cardiology, heart failure and transplantation committee; quality of care and outcomes research and functional genomics and translational biology interdisciplinary working groups; and council on epidemiology and prevention. Circulation. 2006;**113**(14):1807-1816

[7] Elliott P, Andersson B, Arbustini E, Bilinska Z, Cecchi F, Charron P, et al. Classification of the cardiomyopathies: A position statement from the european society of cardiology working group on myocardial and pericardial diseases. European Heart Journal. 2008;**29**(2):270-276

[8] Arbelo E, Protonotarios A, Gimeno JR, Arbustini E, Barriales-Villa R, Basso C, et al. 2023 ESC guidelines for the management of cardiomyopathies: Developed by the task force on the management of cardiomyopathies of the European Society of Cardiology (ESC). European Heart Journal. 2023;**44**(37):3503-3626

[9] Warre S. The pathology of chronic myocarditis. The New England Journal of Medicine. 1933;**208**(11):573

[10] Christian HA. Clinically the myocardium. Archives of Internal Medicine. 1950;**86**(4):491-497

[11] Mattingly TW. The clinical and hemodynamic features of primary myocardial disease. Transactions of the American Clinical and Climatological Association. 1959;**70**:132-141

[12] Blankenhorn MA, Gall EA. Myocarditis and myocardosis; a clinicopathologic appraisal. Circulation. 1956;**13**(2):217-223

[13] Goodwin JF, Gordon H, Hollman A, Bishop MB. Clinical aspects of cardiomyopathy. British Medical Journal. 1961;**1**(5226):675

[14] Goodwin JF, Gordon H, Hollman A, Bishop MB. Idiopathic cardiomegaly. Bulletin of the World Health Organization. 1968;**38**(6):979-992

[15] Goodwin JF, Oakley CM. The cardiomyopathies. British Heart Journal. 1972;**34**:545-552

[16] Maron BJ, Epstein SE. Hypertrophic cardiomyopathy: A discussion of nomenclature. The American Journal of Cardiology. 1979;**43**:1242-1244

[17] Richardson P, McKenna W, Bristow M, et al. Report of the 1995 World Health Organization/international society and Federation of Cardiology Task Force on the definition and classification of cardiomyopathies. Circulation. 1996;**93**(5):841-842

[18] Arbustini E, Narula N, Dec GW, Reddy KS, Greenberg B, Kushwaha S, et al. The MOGE(S) classification for a phenotype-genotype nomen-clature of cardiomyopathy: Endorsed by the world heart federation. Journal of the American College of Cardiology. 2013;**62**(22):2046-2072

[19] Arbustini E, Narula N, Tavazzi L, Serio A, Grasso M, Favalli V, et al. The MOGE(S) classification of cardiomyopathy for clinicians. Journal of the American College of Cardiology. 2014;**64**(3):304-318

[20] Burke MA, Cook SA, Seidman JG, Seidman CE. Clinical and mechanistic insights into the genetics of cardiomyopathy. Journal of the American College of Cardiology. 2016;**68**(25):2871-2886

[21] Villacorta E, Dos-Subirà L, Bermúdez F, González E, Larrañaga J, Limeres J, et al. Comments on the 2023 ESC guidelines for the management of cardiomyopathies. Revista Española de Cardiología (English Ed). 2024;**77**(4):285-289

[22] Argirò A, Ding J, Adler E. Gene therapy for heart failure and cardiomyopathies. Revista Española de Cardiología (English Ed). 2023;**76**(12):1042-1054

[23] Ederhy S, Mansencal N, Réant P, Piriou N, Barone-Rochette G. Role of multimodality imaging in the diagnosis and management of cardiomyopathies. Archives of Cardiovascular Diseases. 2019;**112**(10):615-629

Chapter 2

Cardiomyopathy: Exploring the Causes, Prevention and Management of Cardiomyopathy

Aishwarya Singh, Rohit Mishra and Monika Moni

Abstract

Cardiomyopathies encompass a diverse array of disorders impacting the heart's structure and function. Mutations in genes coding for sarcomeric proteins are linked to various abnormalities that lead to contractile dysfunction and contribute to disease progression. Dilated cardiomyopathy, which can be genetic or acquired, usually manifests with typical heart failure symptoms and reduced ejection fraction. In contrast, restrictive cardiomyopathy is rarer and frequently connected to systemic diseases. Hypertrophic cardiomyopathy can cause exertional dyspnea, atypical chest pain, heart failure, and sudden cardiac death. In arrhythmogenic cardiomyopathy, the hallmark lesion is the replacement of the ventricular myocardium by fibrofatty tissue. Myocardial atrophy occurs progressively with time and manifests with right-sided heart failure and ventricular tachycardia leading to sudden cardiac death. Takotsubo cardiomyopathy is a transient apical ballooning syndrome and stress-induced cardiomyopathy its non-ischemic cardiomyopathy and predominantly affect post-menopausal women. There is transient regional systolic dysfunction of the left ventricle that mimics an acute myocardial infarction but involves only minimal release of cardiac enzymes. The most common clinical presentation in patients with cardiomyopathy is heart failure. While cardiomyopathies can be asymptomatic in their early stages, the symptoms that do appear are usually typical of heart failure.

Keywords: cardiomyopathies, dilated cardiomyopathy, hypertrophic cardiomyopathy, restrictive cardiomyopathy, arrhythmogenic cardiomyopathy, takotsubo cardiomyopathy, systolic dysfunction, diastolic dysfunction, fatty infiltration, Naxos syndrome, broken heart syndrome

1. Introduction

Cardiomyopathies are structural and functional disorders of the myocardium [1]. The pathophysiology of cardiomyopathy involves various mechanisms, including genetic mutations, inflammation, oxidative stress, and neurohormonal dysregulation. These factors contribute to myocardial remodeling, leading to chamber dilation, contractile dysfunction, and eventually heart failure. Cardiomyopathies are a diverse group of myocardial diseases characterized by mechanical and/or electrical dysfunction, typically presenting with abnormal ventricular hypertrophy or dilation. These conditions arise from various causes, often with a genetic component. Depending on the type of cardiomyopathy, heart muscle may become thicker, stiffer, or larger than normal [1]. This can weaken the heart and may cause an arrhythmia or heart failure. Genetic cardiomyopathies are an important cause of HF. Mutations in the sarcomere gene are associated with different types of cardiomyopathy. Cardiomyopathies are driven by both primary conditions of the myocardium and secondary etiologies as part of a multisystem disease. Understanding the pathogenesis of cardiomyopathies comes from identifying the mutations in myocardial proteins involved in energy generation, contraction, cell-to-cell contacts, or connecting the cytoskeleton to the extracellular matrix. This may lead to abnormal contraction and relaxation or dysregulated ion transport that can cause arrhythmia. Genetic predisposition interacts with environmental factors. Genetic testing can help identify specific mutations associated with cardiomyopathy and aid in diagnosis, risk stratification, and family screening [1, 2]. Clinical manifestations of cardiomyopathy range from asymptomatic myocardial dysfunction to heart failure, arrhythmias, and sudden cardiac death. Diagnosis typically involves a combination of clinical evaluation, imaging modalities such as echocardiography and cardiac magnetic resonance imaging, and genetic testing in select cases. Management strategies aim to alleviate symptoms, improve quality of life, and reduce the risk of disease progression. Treatment options include pharmacotherapy, device therapy (e.g., implantable cardioverter-defibrillator), and in selected cases, heart transplantation [2].

2. Types of cardiomyopathies

Cardiomyopathies can be classified according to a variety of criteria including the underlying genetic basis of dysfunction (**Figure 1**) [1].

1. Dilated cardiomyopathy

2. Hypertrophic cardiomyopathy

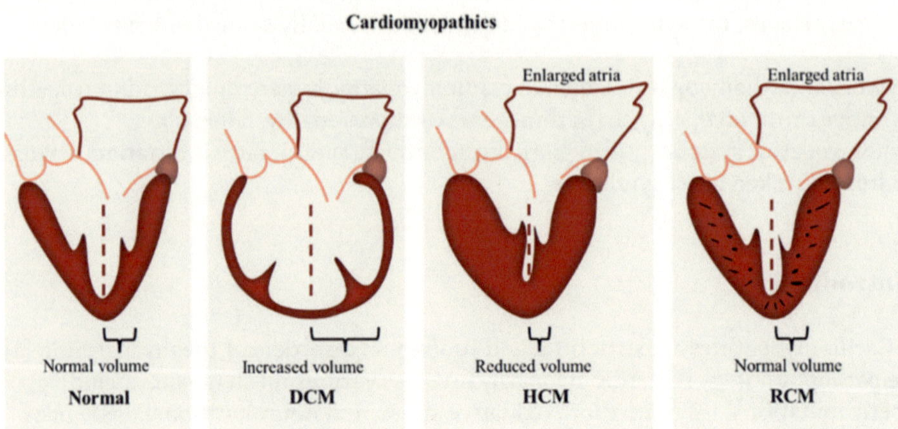

Figure 1.
Scheme demonstrating the morphological features of HCM, DCM, and RCM.

DOI: http://dx.doi.org/10.5772/intechopen.1006610

3. Restrictive cardiomyopathy

4. Arrhythmogenic cardiomyopathy

5. Takotsubo cardiomyopathy

2.1 Dilated cardiomyopathy

Dilated cardiomyopathy (DCM) is a condition affecting the heart muscle, marked by the enlargement and dilation of one or both ventricles, accompanied by reduced contractility, with the left ventricular ejection fraction (LVEF) falling below 40%. Dilated cardiomyopathy (DCM) stems from diverse origins, all impacting ventricular function to different extents [2]. Systolic failure is more prominent than diastolic dysfunction (**Figure 2**). Although symptoms are common among most DCM patients, some may remain asymptomatic due to compensatory mechanisms. However, persistent ventricular enlargement eventually leads to decreased ventricular function, accompanied by conduction abnormalities, ventricular arrhythmias, thromboembolism, and heart failure [2–4].

2.1.1 Causes of dilated cardiomyopathy

1. Infective causes:

- Viral infection—Coxsackie..., HIV, Hepatitis [5–8].

- Parasitic—Trypanosoma cruzi-Chagas disease, toxoplasmosis.

- Spirochete—*Borrelia burgdorferi*—Lyme disease.

- Rikettsial infection—Q fever.

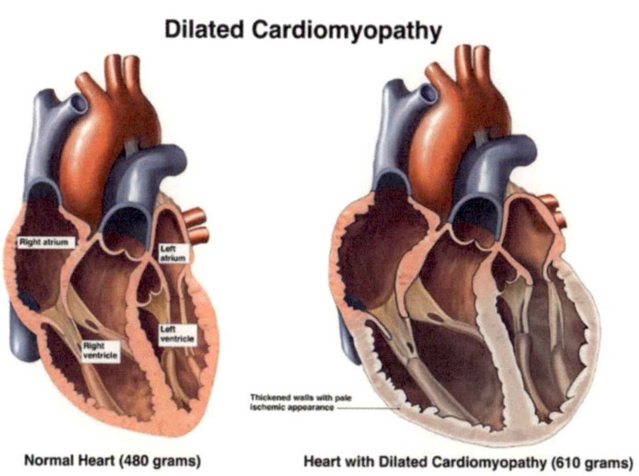

Figure 2.
Comparison between normal heart and heart with dilated cardiomyopathy.

2. Non-infective causes:

    - Granulomatous inflammatory disease: giant cell myocarditis.
    - Polymyositis, dermatomyositis.
    - Collagen vascular disease
    - Transplant rejection

3. Toxic causes:

    - Alcohol
    - Catecholamines: amphetamines, cocaine.
    - Heavy metals: lead, mercury.
    - Occupational exposure: hydrocarbons, arsenicals.
    - Other therapeutic agents: hydroxychloroquine, chloroquine.

4. Metabolic causes:

    - Nutritional deficiency: thiamine, selenium.
    - Electrolyte deficiency: calcium, phosphate, magnesium.
    - Endocrinopathy: thyroid disease, diabetes, central adiposity.

5. Familial causes:

    - Skeletal and cardiac myopathy.
    - Duchenne's dystrophy.
    - Becker's dystrophy.
    - Mitochondrial myopathy.

2.1.2 Management

- EKG shows LVH [9, 10].
- Echocardiography shows an enlarged ventricular chamber, normal or decreased wall thickness, and systolic dysfunction.
- Beta-blockers and angiotensin-converting enzyme inhibitors (ACEIs), ARB are used in ACEI intolerance.

- Diuretics are also used for symptomatic relief and functional status improvement.
- Latest antidiabetic medications (SGLT2 inhibitors) have been shown to improve cardiac function regardless of the presence of diabetes.
- Cardiac resynchronization therapy is a non-pharmacologic treatment option for suitable patients exhibiting dyssynchrony and experiencing persistent symptoms of NYHA class III or IV heart failure despite receiving optimal medical therapy.
- Heart transplantation may be required depending on the severity of symptoms.
- Salt restriction, smoking cessation, obesity management, etc.

2.2 Hypertrophic obstructed cardiomyopathy

HCM, inherited dominantly, presents as left ventricular hypertrophy, often affecting the interventricular septum. End-diastolic wall thickness typically reaches around 15 mm, and there is a heightened risk of sudden cardiac death (SCD) and dynamic obstruction of the left ventricular outflow tract (LVOTO) (**Figure 3**). HCM causes primarily diastolic dysfunction, systolic function is usually preserved [4, 11].

2.2.1 Causes of hypertrophic obstructed cardiomyopathy

HCM is caused by mutations in any one of several genes that encode sarcomere protein. Mutations causing HCM are found most commonly in the genes encoding myosin-binding protein C (MYBP-C) or β-myosin heavy chain (β-MHC/MYH7) followed by genes coding for cardiac TnI, TnT, and α-tropomyosin [7, 8].

2.2.2 Management

- Important cause of sudden cardiac death in sports/athletic players while playing [9, 10].

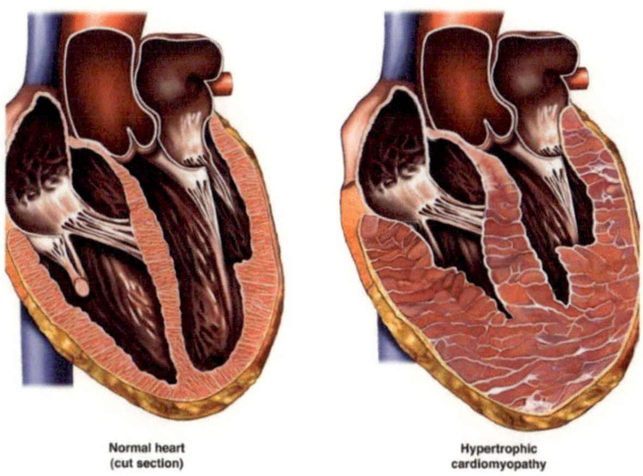

Figure 3.
Comparison between normal heart and heart with hypertrophic cardiomyopathy.

- EKG should be performed to check for arrythmias.
- Echocardiography shows enlarged ventricular chamber, normal or decreased wall thickness, systolic dysfunction.
- First-line treatment for HOCM is beta-blockers, and calcium channel blockers may also be used.
- ACE inhibitors and nitrates should be avoided because they may reduce afterload, potentially worsening left ventricular outflow tract obstruction.
- Septal myectomy is the treatment of choice in young healthy patients.
- Surgical intervention is reserved for patients who are resistant to lifestyle and medical management.

2.3 Restrictive cardiomyopathy

RCM is defined by elevated ventricular filling pressures resulting from a rigid myocardium. Diastolic volumes may be reduced or remain within normal ranges, while systolic function is maintained during the initial phases of the condition. Due to this, the ventricles fail to relax properly and do not fill with enough blood to be pumped to the rest of the body (**Figure 4**) [4, 12].

2.3.1 Causes of restrictive cardiomyopathy

1. Infiltrative: (between myocytes)

    - Amyloidosis [7, 8]:

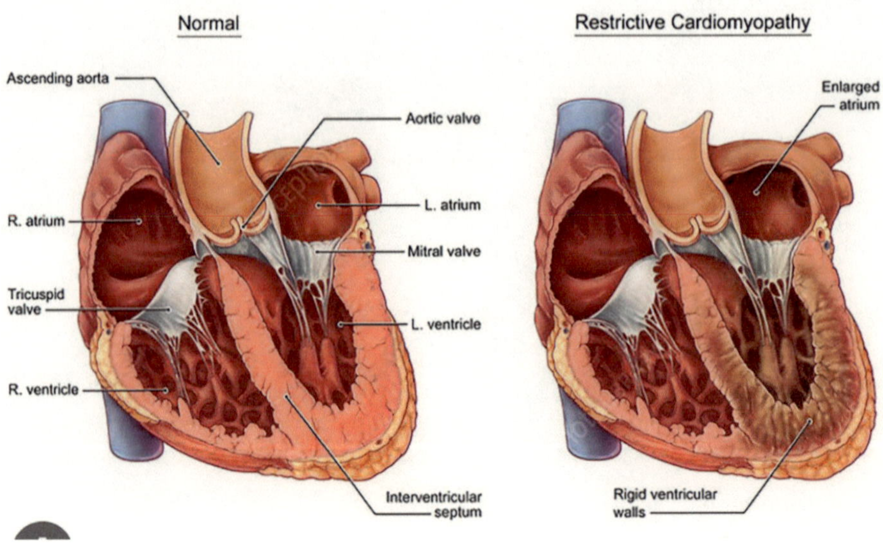

Figure 4.
Comparison between normal heart and heart with restrictive cardiomyopathy.

DOI: http://dx.doi.org/10.5772/intechopen.1006610

- o Primary (light chain amyloid)
- o Secondary (abnormal transthyretin)
- o Senile (normal transthyretin or atrial peptide)

2. Storage: (within myocytes):
    - Hemochromatosis
    - Inherited metabolic defect: Fabry's disease, Glycogen storage disease ii, iii.
3. Fibrotic:
    - Radiation
    - Scleroderma
4. Endomyocardial
    - Tropical endomyocardial Fibrosis
    - Hypereosinophilic response (Loffler's endocarditis)
    - Carcinoid syndrome

2.3.2 Management

- Serum iron studies, autoimmune workup, viral Serologies, serum protein electrophoresis, EKG, Exercise tolerance testing, and, very rarely, biopsies may be needed to diagnose [9, 10].
- Currently, there is no cure for restrictive cardiomyopathy (RCM), but treatments are available to manage the disease's symptoms.
- Diuretics are commonly used to alleviate heart failure symptoms by reducing volume overload, but they must be carefully monitored to avoid excessive diuresis, as patients with RCM depend on high filling pressures to sustain cardiac output.
- Beta-blockers or calcium channel blockers may be used to prolong filling time.
- For hemochromatosis, therapeutic phlebotomy is the preferred treatment.
- In cases of advanced heart failure, options such as cardiac transplantation or left ventricular assist devices may be considered for some patients.

2.4 Arrhythmogenic cardiomyopathy

ARVC is a cardiomyopathy which affects both ventricles, but particularly the right ventricle. The hallmark lesion is the replacement of the ventricular myocardium with fibrofatty tissue, which leads to progressive myocardial atrophy over time, beginning from the epicardium and extending inward toward the endocardium to become transmural, resulting in progressive wall thinning. It is an autosomal dominant disorder that classically manifests with right-sided heart failure and rhythm disturbances, especially ventricular tachycardia, leading to sudden cardiac death, particularly in young patients and athletes (**Figure 5**). The right ventricle wall is severely attenuated due to loss of myocytes, accompanied by massive fatty infiltration and focal fibrosis (**Figure 6**) [13, 14]. Various desmosomal genes have been identified associated with ARVC plakoglobin, desmoplakin, plakophilin-2, desmoglen-2, desmocollin-2 along with TGFβ, and TMEM43.

Naxos syndrome is a disorder characterized by arrhythmogenic cardiomyopathy and hyperkeratosis of planter and palmer skin surfaces and is also associated with plakoglobin mutation [7, 14].

2.4.1 Management

- The diagnosis of AC is often difficult to make. Long-term Holter monitoring is advised [9, 10].
- Once the diagnosis is made, medical therapy such as beta-blockers and antiarrhythmics are started to reduce the instances of arrhythmias.
- Cardiac transplantation may be needed for patients with severe right ventricle abnormalities.
- First-degree relatives should also be tested for the condition.

2.5 Takotsubo cardiomyopathy

Takotsubo cardiomyopathy, also referred to as transient apical ballooning syndrome, apical ballooning cardiomyopathy, stress-induced cardiomyopathy, stress cardiomyopathy, or broken-heart syndrome, is a type of non-ischemic cardiomyopathy

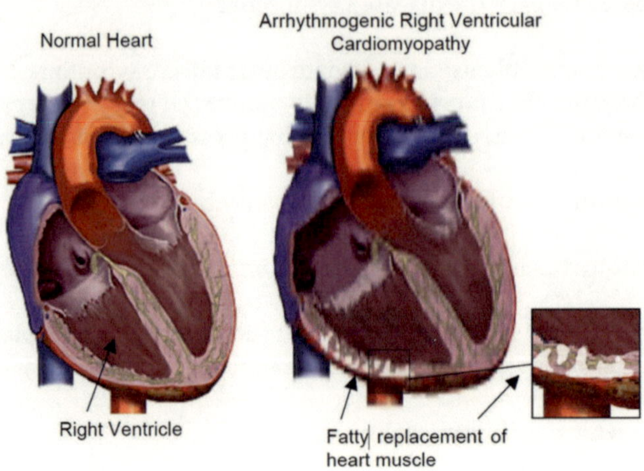

Figure 5.
Comparison between normal heart and heart with arrythmogenic right ventricular cardiomyopathy.

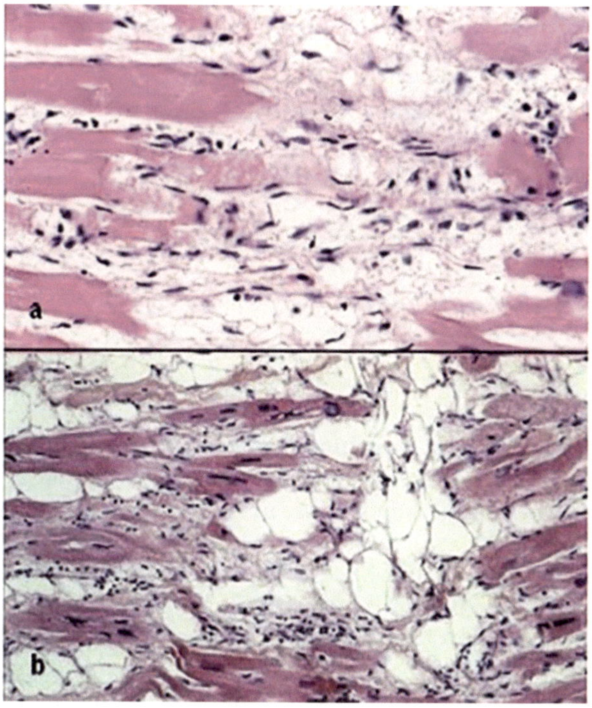

Figure 6.
Histological features of arrhythmogenic right ventricular cardiomyopathy (a) ongoing myocyte death (b) early fibrosis and myocyte death.

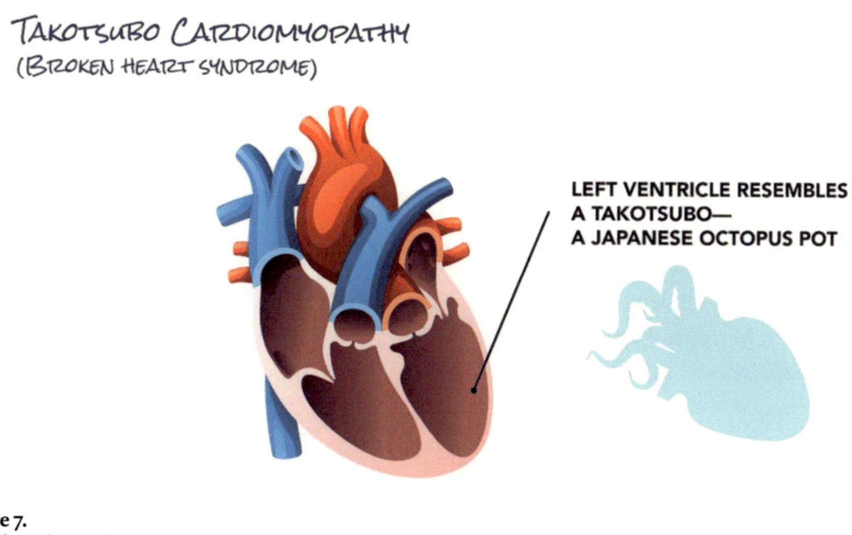

Figure 7.
The tokotsubo cardiomyopathy.

that primarily affects post-menopausal women [15]. It is characterized by temporary regional systolic dysfunction of the left ventricle mimicking acute myocardial infarction but with only minimal release of cardiac enzymes [15, 16]. The term takotsubo means octopus trap in Japanese (**Figure 7**). It has a shape resembling the apical ballooning appearance of the left ventricle during systole [16].

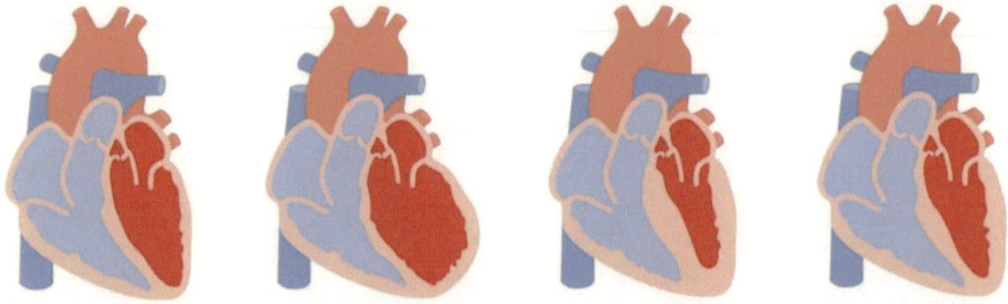

Figure 8.
Schematic diagram showing normal heart with various cardiomyopathy.

The pathophysiological process behind takotsubo cardiomyopathy is still not completely understood. There are various theories, including increased levels of stress-related hormones like catecholamines in the bloodstream, issues with small blood vessels in the heart, inflammation, lack of estrogen, spasms in the larger coronary arteries, and even a type of heart attack that does not fully develop [15]. Catecholamines can lead to microvascular spasms, dysfunction, myocardial stunning, or direct injury to the myocardium. Estrogen provides protective effects for the cardiovascular system, such as promoting vasodilation, guarding against atherosclerosis, and preventing endothelial dysfunction [16]. Consequently, post-menopausal women experience heightened vasoconstriction, impaired endothelium-dependent vasodilation, and increased sympathetic activation in response to psychosocial stress [15, 16].

2.5.1 Management

- EKG should be performed to check for arrhythmia [15, 16].
- Cardiac enzymes should be checked.
- Echo should be performed.
- Medical management includes dual platelet therapy, anti-coagulants, beta-blockers, ACE/ARB, and statins.

Various schematic diagrams showing different morphological features of cardiomyopathies (**Figure 8**) [17].

DOI: http://dx.doi.org/10.5772/intechopen.1006610

Author details

Aishwarya Singh[1], Rohit Mishra[1*] and Monika Moni[2]

1 Department of Pathology, Lincoln American Univerity, Georgetown, Guyana

2 The Christ Hospital, Cincinnati, OH, USA

*Address all correspondence to: sonurohit19@gmail.com

References

[1] Hassoun R, Budde H, Mügge A, Hamdani N. Cardiomyocyte dysfunction in inherited cardiomyopathies. International Journal of Molecular Sciences. 2021;**22**(20):11154. DOI: 10.3390/ijms222011154

[2] Mahmaljy H, Yelamanchili VS, Singhal M. Dilated cardiomyopathy. In: StatPearls. Treasure Island (FL): StatPearls Publishing; 2024. Available from: https://www.ncbi.nlm.nih.gov/books/NBK441911/

[3] Brieler J, Breeden MA, Tucker J. Cardiomyopathy: An overview. American Family Physician. 2017;**96**(10):640-646

[4] National Heart, Lung, and Blood Institute. Cardiomyopathy | NHLBI, NIH [Internet]. www.nhlbi.nih.gov. 2022. Available from: https://www.nhlbi.nih.gov/health/cardiomyopathy

[5] Canepa M, Strait JB, Abramov D, Milaneschi Y, AlGhatrif M, Moni M, et al. Contribution of central adiposity to left ventricular diastolic function (from the Baltimore longitudinal study of aging). The American Journal of Cardiology. 2012;**109**(8):1171-1178. DOI: 10.1016/j.amjcard.2011.11.054. Epub 2012 Jan 17

[6] Canepa M, Strait JB, Milaneschi Y, AlGhatrif M, Ramachandran R, Makrogiannis S, et al. The relationship between visceral adiposity and left ventricular diastolic function: Results from the Baltimore Longitudinal Study of Aging. Nutrition, Metabolism and Cardiovascular Diseases. 2013;**12**(23):1263-1270

[7] Robbins Textbook 10th edition

[8] Loscalzo J, Fauci AS, Kasper DL, Hauser SL, Longo DL, Jameson JL, Harrison TR. Harrison's principles of internal medicine. New York: McGraw-Hill Education; 2021

[9] Sattar Y, Siew KSW, Connerney M, Ullah W, Alraies MC. Management of Takotsubo syndrome: A comprehensive review. Cureus. 2020;**12**(1):e6556. DOI: 10.7759/cureus.6556

[10] Wexler RK, Elton T, Pleister A, Feldman D. Cardiomyopathy: An overview. American Family Physician. 2009;**79**(9):778-784

[11] Raj MA, Ranka S, Goyal A. Hypertrophic obstructive cardiomyopathy. In: StatPearls. Treasure Island (FL): StatPearls Publishing; 2024. Available from: https://www.ncbi.nlm.nih.gov/books/NBK430820/

[12] Brown KN, Pendela VS, Ahmed I, et al. Restrictive cardiomyopathy. In: StatPearls. Treasure Island (FL): StatPearls Publishing; 2024. Available from: https://www.ncbi.nlm.nih.gov/books/NBK537234/

[13] Al-Ghamdi BS. Arrhythmogenic Right Ventricular Cardiomyopathy/Dysplasia. 2017. Available from: https://www.semanticscholar.org/paper/Arrhythmogenic-Right-Ventricular-Cardiomyopathy-Al-Ghamdi/1706702389d2ff40c656cb82227205676d32f7cf

[14] Corrado D, Basso C, Daniel P. Judge—Arrhythmogenic Cardiomyopathy. Available from: https://www.ahajournals.org/doi/full/10.1161/circresaha.117.309345#d1e269

[15] Ahmad SA, Brito D, Khalid N, et al. Takotsubo cardiomyopathy. In: StatPearls. Treasure Island (FL): StatPearls Publishing; 2024.

Available from: https://www.ncbi.nlm.nih.gov/books/NBK430798/

[16] Takotsubo Cardiomyopathy [Internet]. SCAI - Seconds Count. 2022. Available from: https://www.secondscount.org/condition/takotsubo-cardiomyopathy

[17] Cardiomyopathy [Internet]. MedTour. 2023. Available from: https://medtour.help/disease/cardiomyopathy/

Chapter 3

Understanding Cardiomyopathy: Epidemiology, Risk Factors, Types, Mechanisms, Diagnosis, Prevention, and Treatment

Manal Smail, Khemraj Rupee, Sunil Rupee, Carlin Hanoman, Abla Ismail, Ernest A. Adeghate, Raphael Singh, Emanuel Cummings, Chris Sawh and Jaipaul Singh

Abstract

Cardiomyopathies (CMPs) encompass a heterogeneous group of cardiac disorders affecting mainly many of the elderly populations globally. Clinical presentation of cardiomyopathy varies among patients, based on the type and severity of the disorder. Preventing cardiomyopathy involves a multifaceted approach. Management strategies for cardiomyopathy encompass a spectrum of interventions. Medications, including beta-blockers, angiotensin-converting enzyme (ACE) inhibitors, diuretics, and anti-arrhythmic drugs, are commonly prescribed to patients. Device implantation, including pacemakers, implantable cardioverter-defibrillators (ICDs), and ventricular-assist devices (VADs), is necessary in some cases. Lifestyle changes, including dietary modifications. Reduction in alcohol consumption, smoking and stress level, weight management, and regular exercise programmes, are essential components of adherence to self-care. Surgical interventions may be considered, including cardiac surgery and, in severe cases, heart transplantation. This review provides a thorough understanding of cardiomyopathy, covering a wide range of crucial aspects, including epidemiology, risk factors, types, subcellular and molecular mechanisms, clinical presentation, diagnostic approaches, treatment modalities, and prevention strategies, a profound understanding of these aspects is essential for healthcare professionals and researchers to enhance patient health care.

Keywords: cardiomyopathy, myocardium, risk factors, epidemiology, development, treatment, prevention

1. Introduction

Cardiomyopathy is a severe medical condition, which can lead to functional impairments and structural abnormalities in the heart muscle. Cardiomyopathy is characterized by a variety of changes, including myocyte hypertrophy [1], interstitial fibrosis which is a key player in cardiomyopathy that involves the excessive deposition of collagen and other extracellular matrix (ECM) components [2], increased oxidative stress, mitochondrial and endothelial dysfunctions, altered myocardial excitation-contraction coupling (ECC) process, necrosis, and remodeling of the myocardium [3]. These pathophysiological alterations further weaken the myocardium and diminish its ability to pump blood efficiently around the body to meet constant demand [4]. Progressively, these processes disrupt the normal architecture of the myocardium, hindering efficient electrical signal conduction and coordinated contraction [5]. These changes lead to cardiomyopathy manifesting in several distinct forms or subtypes, including dilated (DCM), hypertrophic (HCM), restrictive cardiomyopathies (RCM) and arrhythmogenic right ventricular cardiomyopathy (ARVC) being the primary classifications [6]. Each type exhibits specific pathophysiological traits. For example, dilated cardiomyopathy shows ventricular dilation and systolic dysfunction, whereas hypertrophic cardiomyopathy is characterized by myocardial hypertrophy, potential outflow obstruction, and diastolic dysfunction. Likewise, restrictive cardiomyopathy involves stiffening of the myocardium, leading to impaired ventricular filling [7]. Finally, ARVC is related to a group of clinical conditions that are characterized by right ventricular fibrofatty infiltration, with a predominant arrhythmic presentation [6]. Cardiomyopathy contributes markedly to morbidity and mortality worldwide, with an impact that extends from the individual patient to the broader healthcare system [8]. This cardiovascular disease is associated with a reduced quality of life of the patients due to the limitations imposed by heart failure symptoms. As such, cardiomyopathy demands a multidisciplinary approach in diagnosis, management, treatment, and research into its development, making it a focal point for advancing cardiac health and patient healthcare outcomes.

2. Aim of this review

The purpose of this literature review is to synthesize and examine the current state-of-the-art knowledge regarding cardiomyopathy, its epidemiology, risk factors, types, subcellular and molecular mechanisms associated with pathology of development, clinical presentation, diagnostic approaches, treatment modalities, and prevention strategies. The review is also related to clinical implications to contribute to the existing body of literature by providing a comprehensive overview that encapsulates recent findings and perspectives. It seeks to highlight the complexity of cardiomyopathy, underscore the importance of ongoing research in this area, and identify potential areas for future study. The significance of this work lies in its potential to inform and guide clinical practice, enhance patient care, and direct future research endeavors. This literature review is not only a scholarly exploration but also a step towards improving patient outcomes in cardiomyopathy, thereby playing a critical role in the evolution of cardiovascular medicine.

3. Epidemiology and risk factors

In 2021, 2,268,240 cases were reported to develop dilated cardiomyopathy (DCM), the most common subtype of cardiomyopathy, especially in the USA, France, Italy, and the United Kingdom, with the number increasing annually by 2% [6]. Moreover, the burden of cardiac disorder on global health is substantial, with current epidemiological studies reporting its prevalence at approximately 2.5 million individuals in the United States and over a quarter of a million in the United Kingdom, contributing to a worldwide prevalence estimated at 6 million for all subtypes of cardiomyopathy [6, 9]. The actual incidence of cardiomyopathy is potentially higher than what is recorded, due to its asymptomatic progression in a subset of patients, which can lead to a delay in diagnosis. This under-recognition is emphasized by cardiovascular diseases being responsible for an estimated 18 million deaths per year globally, both in developed and low- and middle-income countries. The epidemiological statistic is steadily increasing and to which cardiomyopathy is a significant contributor, as reported by the World Health Organization (WHO) [6, 10]. This pathology exhibits either no age, religious, or ethnic selectivity. Moreover, accurately quantifying the global incidence of pediatric cardiomyopathy presents a complex challenge, compounded by the heterogeneity of healthcare infrastructures and the variable robustness of epidemiological surveillance across different nations. These estimates suggest a global prevalence of 5–10 cases per million children under 18 years old [11], with potential peak incidences that occur in infants under 1 year [12] and adolescents [13]. Like adults, children can face various types of cardiomyopathies, with dilated cardiomyopathy (DCM) dominating at 35–50% of cases, followed by hypertrophic cardiomyopathy (HCM) at 20–30%, ARVC at 15%, and restrictive cardiomyopathy (RCM) at 5–10% [11].

The etiology of cardiomyopathy in adult and pediatric is multifactorial, encompassing an array of risk factors that converge to precipitate this myocardial pathology. Cardiomyopathy is a complex cardiac condition with a multifactorial etiology, involving a range of interconnected risk factors that contribute to its development. **Figure 1** provides a concise visual representation of these diverse contributors, emphasizing their interplay in the pathogenesis of this condition. Risk factors are diverse, and they serve as essential resources for clinicians, researchers, and public health professionals seeking to mitigate the impact on the development of cardiomyopathy. By integrating

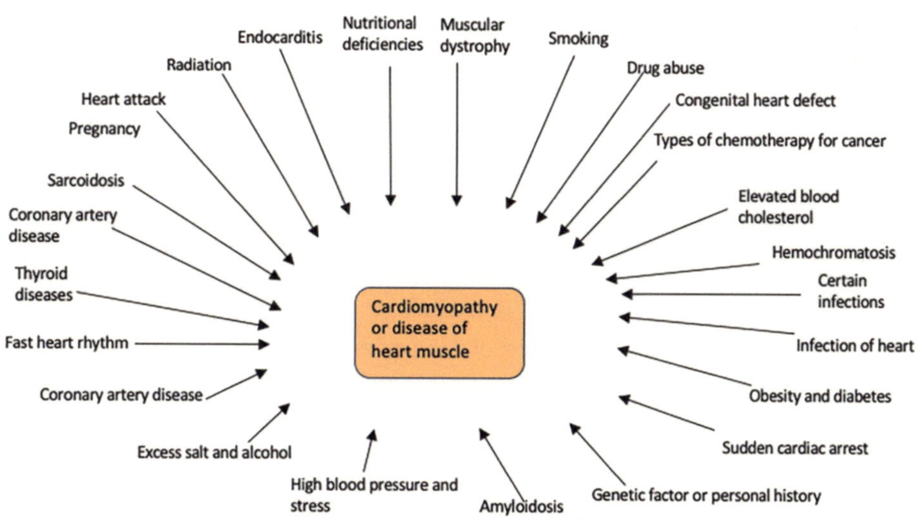

Figure 1.
Diagram illustrating some of the risk factors that are associated with the development of cardiomyopathy or disease of muscle within the heart (drawn by hand).

the latest research findings with clinical insights, this work aims to catalyze the development of advanced management strategies for cardiomyopathy. Ultimately, this endeavor seeks to contribute a substantial and meaningful advancement in the fight against one of the most challenging cardiovascular diseases, thereby fulfilling a critical need in contemporary medical science and patient health care.

4. Subcellular, cellular, and molecular mechanisms

The complexity of cardiomyopathy is further compounded by its multifactorial aetiologies that require a deeper understanding of its varied subcellular, cellular, and molecular dimensions during its development over time. Cellular changes involve remodeling processes that alter the heart muscle's architecture, leading to a compromised contractile apparatus and inefficient cardiac output. One of the critical consequences of cardiomyopathy is heart failure (HF), a condition where the ability of the heart to pump blood effectively is compromised. The progressive loss of cardiomyocytes is due to many pathways related to either necrotic, apoptotic, or autophagic cell death, part of which is highly regulated and programmed [14]. This loss of cellular integrity and function in the heart muscle is a pivotal factor in the progression towards HF, which in itself is a progressive condition originating from myocardial injury due to ischaemia/reperfusion and myocardial infarction due to different health risk and biochemical factors. This injury leads to subcellular and molecular changes manifesting as structural remodeling of cardiomyocytes [15]. This remodeling is characterized by changes in size, shape, and the arrangement of the cells, resulting in impaired contractile function and increased ventricular stiffness, characterized by net accumulation of extracellular matrix proteins in the cardiac interstitial tissues resulting in fibrosis [16, 17]. This, in turn, contributes to both systolic and diastolic dysfunction as in many heart debilitating conditions [16]. One of the key features in this process is the disruption of cardiomyocyte calcium handling via derangement in calcium transporting proteins that in turn, impair the ECC process and contractile function of the heart [18]. Furthermore, oxidative stress leads to increase in reactive oxygen species (ROS) and reactive carbonyl species (RCS) production, coupled with decreased antioxidant defense mechanisms, results in significant mitochondrial and endothelial cell damage resulting in apoptosis [19]. This oxidative stress disrupts the myocardium's force-generating capacity, due to a lack of energy generation by the mitochondria (mitochondrial dysfunction), ultimately, affecting the normal contraction mechanism of the myocardium [20, 21]. Moreover, disruptions in cytoskeletal proteins, such as titin, contribute to myofibrillar disarray and defects in ion channel function contribute to the progressive loss of cardiomyocyte integrity and function [18, 22]. These changes are crucial in understanding the pathophysiology of cardiomyopathy. In terms of genetics, sarcomere mutations play a significant role. It is estimated that 40–60% of cases of hypertrophic cardiomyopathy (HCM) and dilated cardiomyopathy (DCM) have a genetic cause. The mutations associated with these cardiomyopathies often pertain to the regulation of cardiomyocyte contractility. HCM is specifically characterized by pathological left ventricular hypertrophy, myofibril disarrays, and a decrease in myofibril density. These abnormalities lead to a loss of force in isolated cardiomyocytes [23]. Interestingly, patients with HCM may exhibit a higher ejection fraction, not due to increased contractility but rather due to a decrease in ventricular cavity capacity. Conversely, DCM is characterized by a thin and dilated ventricular wall with systolic dysfunction [6]. A mutation in lamin A/C has been linked to the force production in cardiac cells in DCM [24]. The ventricular cavity's volume in DCM patients is substantially larger compared to that in HCM patients, contributing to a significantly lower ejection fraction. The comprehensive flow diagram in **Figure 2** illustrates the intricate cellular and molecular mechanisms underlying the different stages in the development of cardiomyopathy in response to various risk factors, either alone or in combination, resulting in the generation of several intracellular mediators, such as ROS, RCS, inflammation, endothelial and mitochondrial dysfunction, generation of transforming growth factor beta (TGF-β),

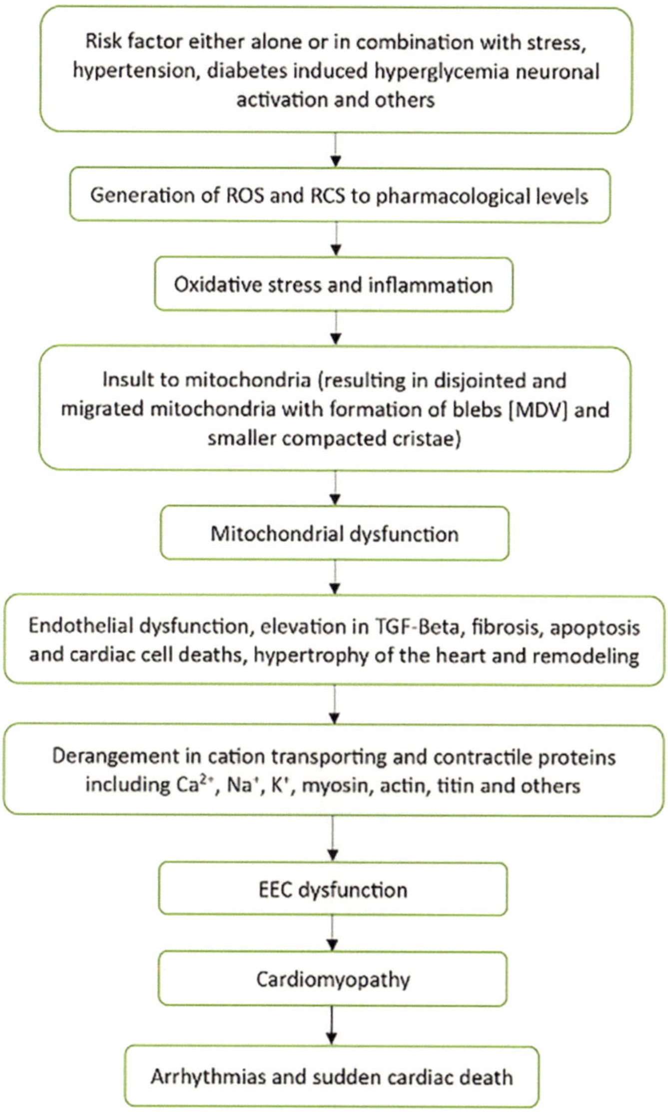

Figure 2.
Flow diagram illustrating the cellular and molecular mechanisms of the development of cardiomyopathy due to insult from risk factors. ROS: reactive oxygen species; ROS = reactive carbonyl species; MDV = mitochondrial-derived vesicles; TGF-β = transforming growth factor beta; Ca^{2+} = calcium; Na^{+} = sodium; K^{+} = potassium (drawn by hand).

fibrosis, apoptosis, cardiac remodeling, and subsequent damage to calcium transporting and contractile proteins, all resulting in impaired cardiac muscle contraction and subsequently, cardiomyopathy and possible sudden cardiac death. This diagram serves as a visual representation of the multifaceted processes involved in the pathogenesis of cardiomyopathy.

5. Types of cardiomyopathies, diagnosis, treatment, and specific management

The flow diagram in **Figure 3** illustrates the different subtypes of known cardiomyopathies to affect patients and they include DCM, HCM, RCM, ARVC and to a lesser extent, left ventricular non-compaction (LVCN) and Takotsubo cardiomyopathy (TCM). The review will now discuss the six types of cardiomyopathies in relation to pathophysiology, treatment, and prevention, but with more emphasis on the first four.

5.1 Dilated cardiomyopathy (DCM)

DCM is characterized by the gradual expansion of the ventricles of the heart, reduced ability to contract, and inadequate filling of the ventricles. The etiology of this condition is complex and arises from a combination of genetic, environmental, and behavioral factors. The complex etiology of DCM is influenced by genetic alterations, viral infections, exposure to toxins, persistent alcohol consumption, autoimmune illnesses, and other risk factors, including hypertension, obesity, and diabetes [6, 25]. DCM is marked by the progressive enlargement of the ventricles of the heart, accompanied with reduced ability to contract to eject blood, and inadequate relaxation delaying filling of the ventricles. The etiology of this condition is complex

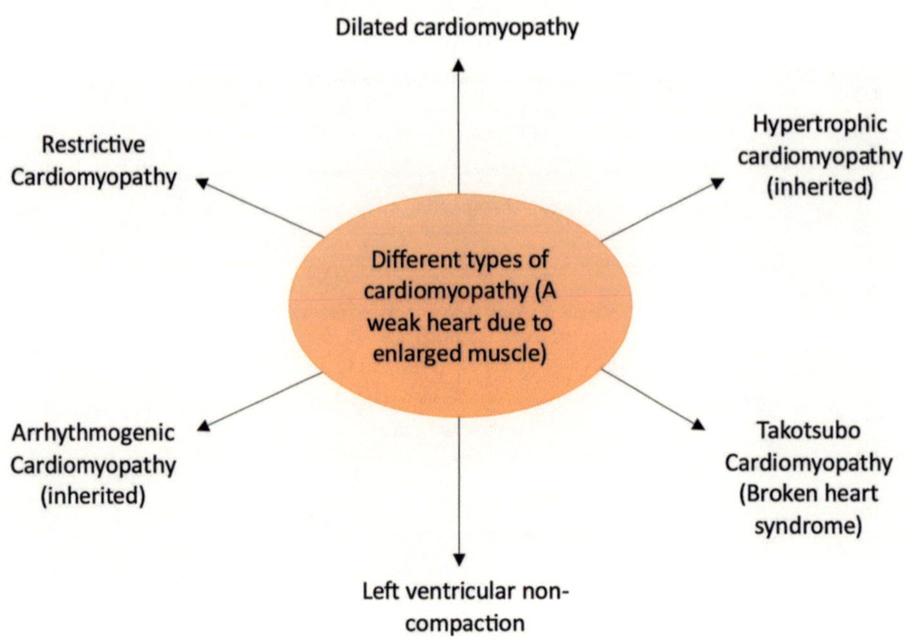

Figure 3.
Flow diagram illustrating the different types of known cardiomyopathies to affect patients (drawn by hand).

and arises from a combination of genetic, environmental, and lifestyle factors [26]. The complex etiology of DCM is influenced by genetic alterations, viral infections, exposure to toxins, persistent alcohol consumption, autoimmune illnesses, and other risk factors, including hypertension, obesity, and diabetes [6, 27].

The pathogenesis of DCM at the subcellular, cellular, and molecular levels includes a variety of structural and functional problems within the myocardium. Myocardial hypertrophy, myofibrillar and mitochondrial disarray including reduced dimensions, apoptosis, fibrosis, and derangements in myocyte calcium and contractile proteins are examples of these [17]. These cellular abnormalities result in reduced contractility and relaxation of the cardiac muscle, leading to decreased pumping capacity and, eventually, heart failure (see **Figure 2**). Furthermore, changes in calcium processing within cardiomyocytes play an important role in contractile failure [18, 22, 28]. Calcium ion dynamics that are out of balance affect normal contraction and relaxation rhythms, further reducing cardiac output. On the molecular level, the pathogenesis of DCM involves complex changes in cardiomyocyte gene expression patterns. These alterations cause disruptions in several signaling pathways that are critical for regular heart function. Among these include anomalies in calcium signaling, β-adrenergic signaling, and stimulation of the renin-angiotensin-aldosterone system (RAAS) [29, 30].

Concurrently, increased reactive oxygen and carbonyl species formation in DCM cause oxidative stress, producing cellular damage and aggravating ventricular contractility dysfunction [19]. A thorough understanding of these molecular pathways is critical for identifying potential therapeutic targets that offer promise for more effective management of this severe disorder [31]. The complex signaling pathways involved in DCM pathophysiology play critical roles in the disease's genesis and progression. Renin-angiotensin-aldosterone system (RAAS) activation is a well-known event in DCM, contributing to cardiac remodeling, fibrosis, and myocardial failure [32]. Another important factor in DCM is dysregulation of β-adrenergic receptors and their related signaling pathways, which results in abnormalities in cardiac function, including contractility and relaxation [30]. Calcium signaling, a critical component of heart function, is severely disrupted in DCM [18]. Calcium homeostasis disruptions inside cardiac cells highlight the development of cardiomyocyte failure, promoting disease progression. A more comprehensive understanding of the functions that these signaling pathways play not only provides insight into the etiology of DCM, but also opens the door to potential treatment strategies [18, 33].

Chronic stress on the heart causes remodeling that includes changes to the molecular, cellular, and extracellular matrix. This remodeling causes changes in the structure, size, and function of the heart, such as ventricular dilatation, decreased contractile function, and increased stiffness [17]. Myocardial remodeling contributes considerably to the development and progression of DCM by inducing cardiac fibrosis, hypertrophy, inflammation, and apoptosis, all of which result in reduced cardiac function and poorer clinical outcomes [17, 34]. The consequences of decreased cardiac output in DCM are systemic, impacting various organs and systems throughout the body. Because the heart's ability to adequately pump blood is impaired, tissue perfusion is reduced, resulting in severe symptoms, such as weariness, weakness, and exercise intolerance. DCM is characterized by pulmonary congestion and oedema, which result from fluid accumulation in the lungs caused by increased pulmonary capillary pressure. Hepatic and renal dysfunctions may occur in severe cases of DCM, as diminished cardiac output limits blood supply to these essential organs, resulting in organ damage [35].

5.2 Diagnosis of DCM

DCM diagnosis is a sophisticated procedure that relies on a thorough examination of clinical symptoms, diagnostic tests, and the meticulous exclusion of other probable causes of heart failure. DCM is characterized clinically by symptoms, such as dyspnoea, tiredness, lower limb oedema, and the presence of an enlarged heart on physical examination. To examine heart function, size, and structural abnormalities, a battery of imaging techniques, including echocardiogram (ECG), cardiac magnetic resonance imaging (MRI), and cardiac computed tomography (CT) scans, are used. Additional laboratory tests, including tests such as as blood analysis and genetic profiles, may also be used to improve diagnostic accuracy. DCM must be distinguished from other cardiomyopathies and cardiac pathologies, such as hypertrophic cardiomyopathy, restrictive cardiomyopathy, ARVC, and ischemic heart disease, with great care [36].

5.3 Treatment of DCM

The treatment of DCM aims to slow disease development, control symptom loads, and improve overall survival. Angiotensin-converting enzyme (ACE) inhibitors, angiotensin receptor blockers (ARBs), beta-blockers, and diuretics are key medications for improving heart function and alleviating symptoms. Devices, such as implantable cardioverter-defibrillators (ICDs) and cardiac resynchronization treatment (CRT), are used in more severe situations to battle arrhythmias and optimize heart function. Heart transplantation emerges as the ultimate option for individuals suffering from end-stage dilated cardiomyopathy who have failed to respond to conventional therapy approaches. The comprehensive care of dilated cardiomyopathy is a complex endeavor that frequently necessitates a multidisciplinary approach that combines medicinal interventions with device-based therapies to improve patient outcomes [37]. While there are recognized therapy techniques such as pharmacological drugs, medical technologies, and heart transplantation, a comprehensive understanding of the disease's pathophysiology is a prerequisite for developing more effective therapeutic strategies. Ongoing research efforts to understand the molecular processes underlying DCM development and identify novel treatment targets have the potential to significantly improve patient outcomes and refine the comprehensive management of this devastating disorder.

5.4 Hypertrophic cardiomyopathy (HCM)

HCM is the most frequent hereditary cardiovascular illness. The condition is caused by mutations in genes that encode cardiac sarcomere protein, resulting in a wide range of phenotypic expressions and clinical outcomes [38]. HCM causes excessive left ventricular (LV) growth (hypertrophy), affecting blood flow [39]. Obstructive HCM is distinguished by a thicker septum that blocks the LV outflow pathway during systole [40]. This obstruction raises intraventricular pressure, lowering cardiac output and causing a cascade of chest discomfort, shortness of breath, and syncope [38]. Non-obstructive HCM has a stiff LV wall, but no major outflow tract blockage. However, this compromises diastolic filling, decreasing cardiac output and producing tiredness, exercise intolerance, and potentially heart failure [39]. Furthermore, myocardial ischemia due to reduced blood supply to the thickened heart muscle can cause chest pain during exercise [38]. Moreover, uncommon, HCM can contribute to this sudden cardiac death in young athletes due to either arrhythmias or LV outflow tract obstruction [38].

5.5 Diagnosis and treatment of HCM

An echocardiogram is normally employed to diagnose hypertrophic cardiomyopathy. The test uses sound waves (ultrasound) to ascertain if the muscle of the heart is enlarged or usually thick. The test also helps to illustrate how well the chambers and valves of the heart are functioning. Other supporting clinical diagnostic tests involve MRI scan (creating analytic images of the heart) and echocardiogram (ECG), especially during exercise stress test to determine irregular heart rhythms and signs of heart thickening [36]. Beta-blockers can be used to lower the heart rate and diminish contractility, relieving chest discomfort and reducing outflow tract blockage [38]. Calcium channel blockers increase diastolic filling in non-obstructive HCM [39]. However, disopyramide directly lowers outflow tract obstruction in obstructive HCM [38]. In extreme situations, surgical myectomy eliminates extra muscle from the septum, enhancing LV performance and easing outflow tract obstruction [38]. Also, lifestyle changes, such as avoiding intense activity, reducing stress, and keeping a healthy weight, are critical for symptom management and long-term well-being [39].

5.6 Restrictive cardiomyopathy (RCM)

RCM is a rare complex subtype of cardiomyopathy characterized by increased myocardial stiffness, which results in poor ventricular filling during diastole and consequent cardiac failure. Unlike other types of cardiomyopathies, which predominantly impact heart contractility, RCM primarily affects the heart's capacity to relax and adequately fill with blood, resulting in decreased cardiac output and the presentation of heart failure symptoms [38]. RCM pathophysiology is essentially characterized by aberrant stiffness and reduced compliance of myocardial tissue. This stiffness can be caused by one of the two things: aberrant substances infiltrating the heart muscle or genetic abnormalities that result in the deposition of abnormal proteins within the myocardium. These structural changes impair normal myocardial architecture and obstruct the heart's relaxation and expansion during diastole, a critical phase for ventricular filling. As a result of RCM, ventricular filling is disturbed, and preload is lowered [41]. Diverse substances, such as amyloid proteins, fibrous tissue, or aberrant mineral deposits like iron, invade the myocardium in infiltrative variants of RCM. These infiltrates alter the normal structure of the myocardium, resulting in increased myocardial stiffness. Genetic variants of RCM, on the other hand, require mutations in specific genes, which are frequently responsible for encoding sarcomere or cytoskeletal proteins. These mutations cause aberrant protein buildup within the heart, worsening cardiac compliance difficulties [42]. RCM causes increased myocardial stiffness, which causes raised filling pressures within the heart chambers, notably in the atria. As a result, the atria widen to handle the higher pressure and compensate for the poor ventricular filling. This compensatory mechanism, however, may eventually fail, resulting in the onset of heart failure symptoms, such as dyspnoea, tiredness, oedema, and exercise intolerance [39].

5.7 Diagnosis and treatment of RCM

Because of the variety of clinical manifestations and the necessity to separate it from other cardiomyopathies, diagnosing restrictive cardiomyopathy can be difficult.

A full clinical assessment, echocardiography, cardiac MRI, and occasionally cardiac biopsy, are used to determine the underlying reason and confirm the diagnosis [40]. RCM management is primarily focused on treating the underlying cause wherever possible. Treatment for infiltrative disorders focuses mostly on managing the underlying condition (e.g., amyloidosis therapy) [43]. Because genetic alterations are typically permanent, the emphasis in genetic RCM often switches to symptom treatment and the prevention of consequences. To relieve symptoms associated with congestion and fluid retention, medications such as diuretics may be administered. Furthermore, the treatment of atrial fibrillation, a prevalent arrhythmia in RCM, and the optimization of heart rate regulation are critical in symptom management [44].

5.8 ARVC

This type of cardiomyopathy is due mainly to the infiltration of fatty materials in the right ventricular free wall of the myocardium. This pathological process arises from the mutation of genes and can cause sudden cardiac death, especially in young people and athletes. This disease is believed to be associated with strenuous exercise and it was first identified and described by Fontaine [45] and is associated with the sudden development of ventricular tachycardia with the left bundle branch pattern [46]. It is believed that 1 in 2500–5000 is affected, accounting for 7–10% of sudden unexplained death in an individual less than 65 years of age. It is very prevalent in young adults and male-to-female ratio of 2.7 to 1 [47, 48]. The precise pathophysiology of ARVC is still unknown, but it is believed to involve apoptosis of cardiomyocytes. Recent studies have identified the Sino-atrial pacemaker channel hyperpolarization activated cyclic nucleotide-gated potassium as the culprit in the pathophysiology of ARVC [49, 50]. It is believed that the disease process initiates in the subepicardial region of the heart, and it then extends to the endocardial region and then spreads transmurally around the myocardium. Some of the symptoms of this cardiac disease are palpitation fatigue, inflammation, syncope, and spontaneous cardiac arrest during strenuous physical activities.

5.9 Diagnosis and treatment of ARVC

Patients are normally diagnosed employing the history of the patient, electrocardiogram, echocardiograph, magnetic resonance imaging (MRI), and endocardial biopsy. The goal of management and treatment of ARVC is to prevent and decrease the number of sudden deaths employing pharmacological agents, and other clinical procedures, such as surgical (cardiac transplant), catheter ablation (to treat incessant tachycardia), and placement of an implantable cardioverter-defibrillator (to prevent sudden cardiac death of the patient) [6, 11].

5.10 Left ventricular non-compaction (LVNC) and Takotsubo cardiomyopathy (TCM)

Left ventricular non-compaction (LVNC) is an unusual, rare type of cardiomyopathy in left ventricular muscle of the heart. In this rare case, the left ventricle muscle develops into two structural forms as smooth and loose, like a thick web. In turn, the loose muscle tends to extend into the left ventricle resulting in weakness of the cardiac ventricular muscle and thereby, preventing the heart from pumping an adequate volume of blood around the body to meet constant demand. LVNC is diagnosed based on several clinical parameters, including cardiac testing with echocardiography, family history, medical history, and physical examination. Diagnosed patients are treated with either an implantable cardioverter-defibrillator (ICD) or a pacemaker (cardiac resynchronization therapy). On the other hand, TCM or broken heart syndrome is also another rare condition that can develop over time due to extreme stress, which results in the heart muscle unable to work efficiently as a pump. TCM occurs in both men, but more so in menopausal women. TCM is diagnosed by chest X-ray, blood biomarkers and tests, cardiac echocardiogram, coronary angiograph or cardiac catheterization and electrocardiogram (ECG test). TCM is treated with several drugs, including ACE inhibitor, beta-blockers, anticoagulants, intravenous fluids, oxygen therapy, and psychotherapy [6, 11].

6. General comments on cardiomyopathy including treatments, management, and prevention strategies

Comprehensive management and prevention of cardiomyopathy involve a multifaceted approach that includes both non-pharmacological and pharmacological strategies, as well as device-based interventions and surgical options when necessary. Cardiomyopathy pathophysiology includes a wide range of causes, demanding customized diagnostic and therapeutic strategies. A better understanding of the underlying mechanisms, as well as a multidisciplinary approach to patient therapy, is essential for properly managing this complex and complicated cardiac disorder. **Figure 3** summarizes the main three forms of treatment of cardiomyopathy, including pharmacological, devices, and surgery. Accurate diagnosis of cardiomyopathy hinges on a multidimensional approach. A comprehensive medical history, family history, and physical examination provide initial insights. Advanced imaging techniques, including echocardiography, cardiac MRI, and nuclear imaging, offer critical structural and functional data. Genetic testing plays a pivotal role in identifying familial cardiomyopathy forms. In select cases, endomyocardial biopsy confirms diagnosis and guides therapeutic decisions [42].

In terms of medical management of cardiomyopathy, **Figure 4** summarizes pharmacological, devices, and surgical intervention, used to manage cardiomyopathy. Pharmacological therapies are tailored to the type of cardiomyopathy and may include antihypertensives, blood thinners, anti-arrhythmic, and cholesterol-lowering medications to address various aspects, such as blood pressure, clot formation, heart rhythm abnormalities, and dyslipidemia [51–54]. Additional treatments might involve aldosterone antagonists and corticosteroids to manage fluid retention and inflammation, respectively [12, 55].

Surgi. For those where medication is insufficient, device-based interventions, such as pacemakers, implantable cardioverter-defibrillators, cardiac resynchronization therapy systems (CRTS), and left ventricular-assist devices (VADs), may be necessary to manage rhythm disorders to improve cardiac output [56–59]. In severe or advanced cases, surgical interventions like septal myectomy or heart transplants become options to consider [60, 61]. Less invasive surgeries like alcohol septal ablation and catheter ablation are also employed for specific complications [62, 63]. These approaches collectively aim to slow disease progression, alleviate symptoms, reduce complications, and improve patient survival and quality of life.

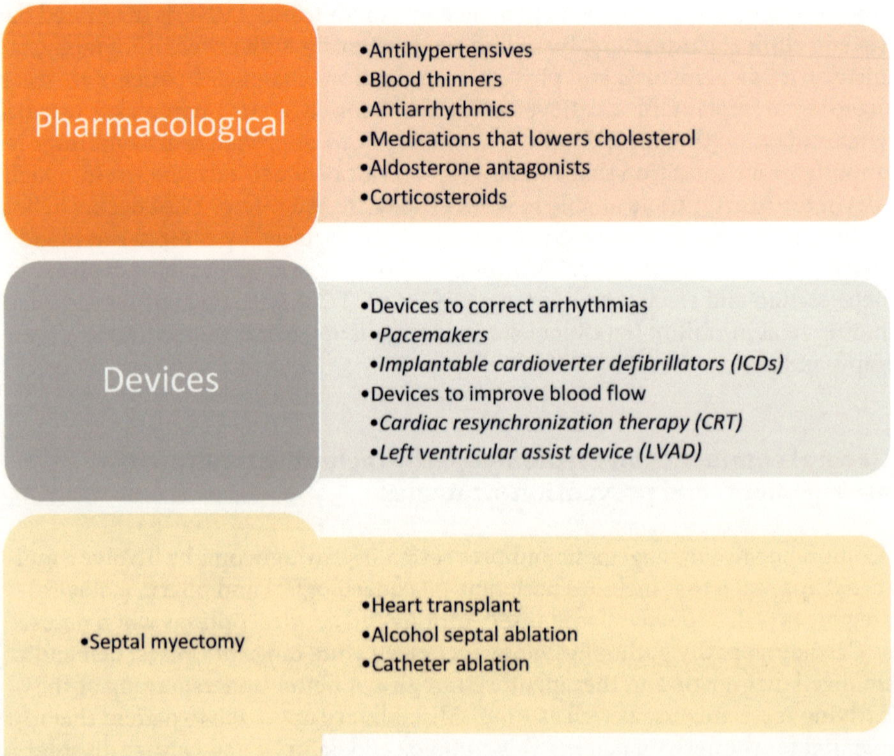

Figure 4.
Diagram illustrating the pharmacological, devices, and surgical intervention, to treat cardiomyopathy (drawn by hand).

7. Genes and cardiomyopathy

Both DCM and HCM are genetic disorders which can lead to heart failure, life-threatening arrhythmia, and subsequently sudden cardiac death (see **Figure 2**) and in these cases, the patients may require either heart transplantation or cardiac device implantation [64, 65]. These cardiomyopathies have prevalence rates of approximately 0.004% and 0.2%, respectively, with familial or genetic-related cases accounting for 20–50% of all cases [64–67]. There are more than 50 genes that are associated with the development of these cardiomyopathies, with some ethnic-specific founder mutations in different parts of the world [68, 69]. Moreover, it has been reported that racial differences can affect mutational profiles with the genetic basis of these disorders different from one ethnic group to another among patients and with some patients with cardiomyopathies showing diverse clinical phenotypes [64], In addition, it has been reported that the phenotypes may correspond to specific genotypes. One typical example is that *LMNA* mutations in DCM patients are linked to a high incidence of sudden cardiac death [70, 71]. Current genetic evidence has indicated that the identification of the genotypes involved in prognosis and treatment response of patients with cardiomyopathy may contribute to risk stratification and accurate treatment decisions by the clinicians. However, further research is warranted in this novel area of study on cardiomyopathy in relation to its development and therapy.

8. Prevention and treatment of cardiomyopathy

Genetic or inherited types of cardiomyopathies are very difficult to prevent but, changes or adopting in lifestyle, including daily moderate exercise, and diet modifications play significant and measurable roles that prevent the development and even progression of cardiomyopathy and they may even cure the disease. The susceptible patient must focus on a nutritious diet low in sodium, fats, and carbohydrates, but high in fruits, fibers, vegetables, and whole grains, foods which are rich in oxidants to manage blood pressure and weight [55]. The American Heart Association (AHA) underscores the importance of a low-fat and low-salt diet for heart health [72]. Regular physical activity, as recommended by the Physical Activity Guidelines for Americans [65], plays a vital role, with a suggestion of at least 150 minutes of moderate aerobic exercise weekly to maintain cardiovascular health. Achieving and maintaining a healthy weight range is crucial as is ensuring adequate sleep and reducing stress. Abstinence from alcohol and tobacco is also advised to minimize cardiac stress [65, 72]. The flow diagram in **Figure 5** illustrates several natural ways whereby people can help themselves to both reduce and prevent the development of cardiomyopathy.

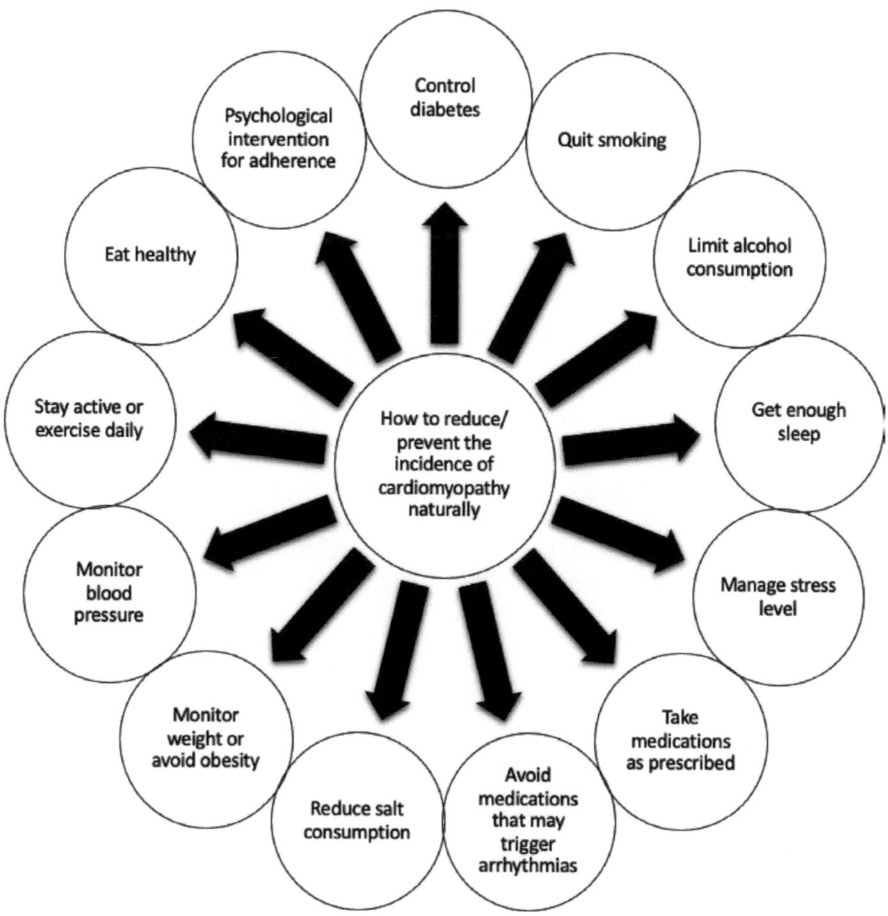

Figure 5.
Diagram illustrating several natural ways whereby people can help themselves to both reduce and prevent the development of cardiomyopathy leading to longevity and a better quality of life (drawn by hand).

They must avoid obesity, control their diabetes or avoiding it, reducing salt, alcohol drinking, smoking habits, and stress levels, monitor their weight and blood pressure regularly, practising yoga and meditation and seek psychological intervention to adhere to daily drug intakes and lifestyle changes [67, 69, 71]. Together, these proposed cost-effective interventions can lead to longevity and a better quality of life.

9. Conclusion

In conclusion, the comprehensive review of cardiomyopathies presented here sheds light on the intricate nature of these cardiac disorders. Cardiomyopathies are a diverse group of conditions affecting both adults and children worldwide, regardless of common cardiovascular comorbidities. The epidemiological data underscore the substantial public health concern, with a prevalence of approximately 1 in 500 adults and an incidence of about 12 cases per million in children. Understanding the risk factors associated with cardiomyopathy is crucial for early identification and prevention. Genetic mutations, family history, viral infections, lifestyle factors, and comorbid conditions contribute to the complexity of the disease, emphasizing the need for personalized management strategies. The review categorizes cardiomyopathies into distinct types, each with its own set of characteristics, which further highlight the complexity of the condition. The subcellular, cellular, and molecular mechanisms underlying cardiomyopathy development elucidate the intricate pathophysiology, providing a foundation for targeted therapeutic interventions and ongoing research. Clinical presentation varies, but based on type and severity, an early and accurate diagnosis is essential for effective management. A combination of diagnostic approaches, including medical history, physical examination, and various imaging and genetic tests, aids in this process. Prevention strategies encompass lifestyle modifications and genetic counseling, emphasizing the importance of healthy habits and managing underlying risk factors. The treatment spectrum includes medications, device implantation, lifestyle changes, and surgical interventions, all tailored to the specific needs of each patient. Emerging therapies like gene therapy hold promise for more targeted approaches. The review also offers healthcare professionals and researchers the knowledge needed to enhance patient care and alleviate the global burden of this intricate cardiac condition. Continued research and advancements in diagnosis and treatment hold hope for improved outcomes for individuals affected by cardiomyopathy.

Author details

Manal Smail[1], Khemraj Rupee[1], Sunil Rupee[1], Carlin Hanoman[1], Abla Ismail[2], Ernest A. Adeghate[3], Raphael Singh[4], Emanuel Cummings[5], Chris Sawh[6] and Jaipaul Singh[1*]

1 School of Pharmacy and Biomedical Sciences, University of Central Lancashire, Preston, England, UK

2 Corniche Hospital, Abu Dhabi, United Arab Emirates

3 Department of Human Anatomy, College of Medicine and Health Sciences, United Arab Emirates University, Al Ain, UAE

4 Department of Chemistry, University of Guyana, Georgetown, Guyana

5 Office of the Vice Chancellor, University of Guyana, Georgetown, Guyana

6 Norfolk and Norwich University Hospital, NHS Foundation Trust, Norwich, England, UK

*Address all correspondence to: jsingh3@uclan.ac.uk

References

[1] Hill JA, Olson EN. Cardiac plasticity. New England Journal of Medicine. 2008;**358**(13):1370-1380

[2] Frangogiannis NG. The extracellular matrix in myocardial injury, repair, and remodelling. Journal of Clinical Investigation. 2017;**127**(5):1600-1612

[3] Heineke J, Molkentin JD. Regulation of cardiac hypertrophy by intracellular signalling pathways. Nature Reviews Molecular Cell Biology. 2006;7(8):589-600

[4] Dorn GW 2nd. Apoptotic and non-apoptotic programmed cardiomyocyte death in ventricular remodelling. Cardiovascular Research. 2009;**81**(3):465-473

[5] Camelliti P, Borg TK, Kohl P. Structural and functional characterization of cardiac fibroblasts. Cardiovascular Research. 2005;**65**(1):40-51

[6] Global Data. Cardiomyopathies Epidemiology Analysis and Forecast, 2021-2031. Report Code GDHCER296-22-ST. 2022. Available from: https://www.globaldata.com/store/report/cardiomyopathies-epidemiology-analysis/

[7] Maron BJ, Ommen SR, Semsarian C, Spirito P, Olivotto I, Maron MS. Hypertrophic cardiomyopathy: Present and future, with translation into contemporary cardiovascular medicine. Journal of the American College of Cardiology. 2020;**75**(1):83-99

[8] Abbate A, Biondi-Zoccai GG, Bussani R, et al. Myocardial cell death in heart failure: A pathophysiological review and potential implications for therapy. American Journal of Cardiovascular Drugs. 2006;**6**(4):257-267

[9] McNally EM, Ackerman MJ. An update on genetic cardiomyopathies. Circulation. 2015;**131**(1):26-37

[10] World Health Organization. Cardiovascular Diseases. 2023. Available from: https://www.who.int/health-topics/cardiovascular-diseases [Accessed: January 28, 2024]

[11] Kaynak-Yılmaz Ö, Tayfur P, Ergüven M. Paediatric cardiomyopathy: Current state of knowledge and future directions. World Journal of Cardiology. 2020;**12**(1):15-28

[12] Seiler C, Maisch B, Siegmund A, Beer G. Epidemiology of childhood cardiomyopathy. Archives of Disease in Childhood. Heart. 2017;**102**(5):406-410

[13] Asimaki A, Tandri H, Duffy ER, et al. Hypertrophic cardiomyopathy: Molecular mechanisms and clinical management. Circulation Research. 2020;**126**(4):556-568

[14] Chen YJ, Chien CS, Chiang CE, et al. From genetic mutations to molecular basis of heart failure treatment: An overview. International Journal of Molecular Sciences. 2021;**22**(12):Article 6617

[15] Whelan RS, Kaplinski V, Kitsis PN. Cell death in pathogenesis of heart diseases: Mechanisms and significances. Annual Review of Physiology. 2010;**72**:19-44

[16] Pong K, Christia P, Frangogiannis NG. The pathogenesis of cardiac fibrosis. Cellular and Molecular Life Sciences. 2015;**71**(4):549-574

[17] D' Souza A, Howarth CF, Yanni J, Dobrzynski H, Boyett MN,

Adeghate E, et al. Chronic effect of mild hyperglycaemia on left ventricle transcriptional profile and structural remodelling in the spontaneously type 2 Goto-Kakizaki rat. Heart Failure Review. 2014;**19**:65-74. DOI: 10.107/s10741-013-9376-9

[18] Rupee S, Rupe K, Singh RB, Hanoman C, Smail M, Singh J. Diabetes-induced chronic heart failure is due to defects in calcium transporting and regulatory contractile proteins: Cellular and molecular evidence. Heart Failure Review. 2022;**28**(3):627-644. DOI: 10.1007/s10741-022-10271-5

[19] Alomar FA, Al-Rubaish A, Al-Muhanna F, Al-Ali AA, McMillan JE, Singh J, et al. Adeno-associated viral transfer of glyoxalase-1 blunts carbonyl and oxidative stress in heart of type 1 diabetic rats. Antioxidants. 2020;**9**(7):Article 592 (22 pages). DOI: 10.3390/antiox9070592

[20] Mann DL, Bristow MR. Mechanisms and models in heart failure. Circulation. 2005;**111**(21):2837-2849

[21] Ingles J, Sarina T, Yeates L, et al. Clinical predictors of genetic testing outcomes in hypertrophic cardiomyopathy. Genetics in Medicine. 2018;**20**(9):972-977

[22] Smail MM, Ismael AB, Howarth FC, Adeghate E, Singh RB, Bidasee K, et al. Titin protein and its role in the pathophysiology of heart failure: A mini review. World Heart Journal. 2022;**14**:1-20

[23] McNally EM, Mestroni L. Dilated cardiomyopathy: Genetic determinants and mechanisms. Circulation Research. 2017;**121**(7):731-748

[24] Vikhorev PG, Vikhoreva NN. Cardiomyopathies and related changes in contractility of human heart muscle. International Journal of Molecular Sciences. 2018;**19**(8):2234

[25] Taylor MR, Roberts WC, Mason JW. Pathophysiology of heart failure. Circulation. 2019;**139**(15):1909-1925

[26] Frustaci D, Chimenti S, Cihakova K, et al. ESC guidelines for the diagnosis and management of takotsubo cardiomyopathy. European Heart Journal. 2021;**42**(3):319-357

[27] Hershberger RE, Morales A, Kong Y, Li D. Dilated cardiomyopathy: The role of genetic factors. Circulation Research. 2020;**112**(11):1563-1573

[28] Frey N, Katus HA. Myocardial fibrosis in heart failure: A new paradigm for understanding pathogenesis and developing therapies. Circulation Research. 2009;**105**(1):17-24

[29] Luo W, Grueter CE, Rao V, et al. Disruption of calcium cycling and PLB regulation by Galphaq in human dilated cardiomyopathy. Circulation Research. 2008;**103**(10):1043-1045

[30] Zhang Y, Yang Z, Yani J, Qureshi MA, Logantha SJ, Kassab S, et al. Electrical conduction system remodelling in streptozotocin-induced diabetes mellitus rat heart. Frontiers in Physiology. 2019;**10**:Article 826

[31] Madesh M, Balasubramanian N. Role of oxidative stress in the pathogenesis of dilated cardiomyopathy. Clinical and Experimental Pharmacology and Physiology. 2017;**44**(8):709-716

[32] Ferrairo CM. Cardiac remodelling and RAS inhibition. Therapeutics Advances in Cardiovascular Diseases. 2016;**10**(3):162-171

[33] Chen W, Zhang R, Zhang X, et al. Role of renin-angiotensin-aldosterone system in regulating cardiac remodelling and fibrosis in dilated cardiomyopathy. Journal of Translational Medicine. 2020;**18**(1):Article 76

[34] Seidman CE, Seidman JG. Genetics of dilated cardiomyopathy: Molecular basis and clinical implications. Journal of Clinical Investigation. 2017;**127**(8):2783-2791

[35] Maron BJ, McKenna WJ, Spirito NP, et al. Recommendations for evaluation and management of hypertrophic cardiomyopathy in adults. Journal of the American College of Cardiology. 2020;**75**(24):3006-3079

[36] Felker G, Seidman MA, McKenna WJ. Dilated cardiomyopathy: Genetic causes, clinical manifestations, and therapeutic options. Circulation Research. 2009;**104**(7):1004-1013

[37] Ponikowski P, Voors AW, Anker SD, et al. ESC guidelines for the diagnosis and management of acute and chronic heart failure. European Heart Journal. 2016;**37**(27):2129-2200

[38] Maron BJ, Spirito MJ, Ackerman MJ. Hypertrophic cardiomyopathy. In: Braunwald's Heart Disease: A Textbook of Cardiovascular Medicine. Philadelphia, PA: Elsevier. Chapter 49

[39] Elliott PM, Maron BJ, McKenna WJ, et al. ESC guidelines for the diagnosis and management of hypertrophic cardiomyopathy. European Heart Journal. 2014;**35**(39):2733-2779

[40] Ommen SR, Michels M, Mahmod SS, et al. Myocardial fibrosis in hypertrophic cardiomyopathy: New insights from imaging and tissue studies. Nature Reviews Cardiology. 2020;**17**(12):729-744

[41] Schaefer TJ, McKenna WJ, Maron BJ, et al. Contemporary diagnosis and management of restrictive cardiomyopathy. Circulation Heart Failure. 2015;**8**(6):759-775

[42] McKenna WJ, Elliott P, Spirito NP, et al. Diagnosis of hypertrophic cardiomyopathy. British Heart Journal. 2006;**77**(6):570-589

[43] Gertz MA, Dispenzieri A, Kyle RA, et al. Treatment of cardiac amyloidosis. Nature Reviews Cardiology. 2016;**13**(8):495-508

[44] Yancy CW, Jessup M, Bozkurt E, et al. 2016 ACC/AHA/HFSA heart failure clinical practice guidelines. Circulation. 2016;**134**(4):e136-e435

[45] Basso C, Corrado D, Marcus FI, Nava A, Thiene G. Arrhythmogenic right ventricular cardiomyopathy. Lancet. 2009;**373**(9671):1289-1300

[46] Wichter T, Borggrefe M, Breithardt G. Arrhythmogenic right ventricular cardiomyopathy. Aetiology, diagnosis, and therapy. Medizinische Klinik (Munich, Germany). 1998;**93**(4):268-277

[47] Shah SN, Umapathi KK, Olivert. arrhythmogenic right ventricular cardiomyopathy. National Library Medicine. In: StatPearls [Internet]. Treasure Island (FL), USA: StatPearls Publishing; 2023. Available from: https://www.ncbi.nlm.nih.gov/books/NBK470378/

[48] Tsang CD, Link MS. Sudden cardiac deaths in athlete. Texas Heart Institute Journal. 2012;**48**(4):Article e207513

[49] D'Souza A, Wang Y, Anderson C, et al. A circadian clock in the sinus node mediates day-night rhythms in

Hcn4 and heart rate. Heart Rhythm. 2021;**18**(5):801-810

[50] Anderson C, Forte G, Hu W, Zhang H, Boyett MR, D'Souza A. Non-canonical role of the sympathetic nervous system in the day-night rhythm in heart rate. Philosophical Transactions of the Royal Society B - Journals. 2023;**378**(1879). Article 2022017

[51] Lee G, Tiano AV, Low SW, et al. Pharmacological approaches in the treatment and management of cardiomyopathies. Pharmacology & Therapeutics. 2018;**185**:34-48

[52] Lip GYH, Coca A, Kahan T, et al. Hypertension and cardiac arrhythmias: Executive summary of a consensus document from the European Heart Rhythm Association (EHRA) and ESC Council on Hypertension, endorsed by the Heart Rhythm Society (HRS), Asia-Pacific Heart Rhythm Society (APHRS) and Sociedad Latino Americana de Estimulación Cardíaca y Electrofisiología (SOLAECE). European Heart Journal - Cardiovascular Pharmacotherapy. 2015;**1**(2):96-111

[53] Calkins H, Kuck KH, Cappato R, et al. 2022 HRS/EHRA/ECAS/APHRS/SOLAECE expert consensus statement on catheter and surgical ablation of atrial fibrillation. Heart Rhythm. 2022;**19**(10):e275-e444

[54] Grundy SM, Stone NJ, Bailey AL, et al. 2018 a guideline on the management of blood cholesterol. Journal of the American College of Cardiology. 2018;**73**(24):e285-e350

[55] O'Donnell MJ, Chin SL, Rangarajan S, et al. Global and regional effects of potentially modifiable risk factors associated with acute stroke in 32 countries (INTERSTROKE): A case-control study. The Lancet. 2015;**386**(9990):761-775

[56] Brugada J, Katritsis DG, Arbelo E, et al. 2013 ESC guidelines on cardiac pacing and cardiac resynchronization therapy. European Heart Journal. 2013;**34**(29):2281-2329

[57] Kléber AG, Janse MJ, Wilms-Schopman FJG, et al. Changes in conduction velocity during acute ischemia in ventricular myocardium of the isolated porcine heart. Circulation. 1997;**95**(3):684-691

[58] Auerbach DS, Grzda KR, Furspan PB, et al. Structural heterogeneity promotes triggered activity, reflection, and arrhythmogenesis in cardiac tissue. Journal of Molecular and Cellular Cardiology. 2014;**74**:48-57

[59] Kirk EW, Gold MR, Kutyifa V, et al. The evolving role of cardiac resynchronization therapy in reducing mortality and heart failure hospitalization in the post-ACCORDION era. Journal of the American College of Cardiology. 2020;**75**(11):1297-1308

[60] Maron MS, Rowin EJ, Maron BJ, et al. Contemporary natural history and management of nonobstructive hypertrophic cardiomyopathy. JAMA Cardiology. 2020;**5**(4):419-428

[61] Taylor DM, Batten LA, Brandie JW, et al. The role of artificial intelligence in the diagnosis and management of cardiomyopathy. Journal of Cardiac Failure. 2023;**29**(1):54-64

[62] Kotecha D, Piccini JP, Mohan R, et al. Atrial fibrillation in heart failure: What should we do? European Heart Journal. 2020;**41**(48):4515-4527

[63] Gómez-Outes E, Terleira-Fernández AI, Suárez-Gea ML, Vargas-Castrillón E. Anticoagulant therapy in atrial fibrillation and heart failure. New England Journal of Medicine. 2023;**388**(6):474-485

[64] Tobita T, Nomura S, Fugita T, et al. Genetic basis of cardiomyopathy and the genotypes involved in prognosis and left ventricular reverse remodelling. Scientific Report. 2018;**8**:Article 1998

[65] American Heart Association. American Heart Association Recommendations for Physical Activity in Adults and Kids. 2020. Available from: https://www.heart.org/en/healthy-living/fitness/fitness-basics/aha-recs-for-physical-activity-in-adults [Accessed: January 28, 2024]

[66] Maron BJ. Hypertrophic cardiomyopathy: A systematic review. JAMA. 2002;**287**:1308-1320

[67] Garcia MJ, McNamara PM, Gordon T, Kannell WB. Morbidity and mortality in diabetics in the Framingham population. Diabetes. 1974;**23**(2):105-111

[68] McNally EM, Golbus JR, Puckelwartz MJ. Genetic mutations and mechanisms in dilated cardiomyopathy. Journal of Clinical Investigation. 2013;**123**:19-26

[69] Johnson NB, Hayes LD, Brown K, et al. CDC National Health Report: Leading causes of morbidity and mortality and associated behavioural risk and protective factors—United States, 2005-2013. MMWR Supplements. 2014;**63**(4):3-27

[70] Becane HM et al. High incidence of sudden death with conduction system and myocardial disease due to Lamins A and C gene mutation. PACE. 2000;**23**:1661-1666

[71] Martinus R, Corban R, Wackerhage H, et al. Effect of psychological intervention on exercise adherence in type 2 diabetic subjects. Annals of the New York Academy of Sciences. 2006;**1084**:350-360

[72] Smith SC, Benjamin EJ, Bonow RO, et al. AHA/ACC/AACVPR/AAPA/ABC/ACPM/ADA/AGS/APhA/ASPC/NLA/PCNA guideline for the prevention, detection, evaluation, and management of high blood pressure in adults. Journal of the American College of Cardiology. 2018;**71**(19):e127-e248

Chapter 4

Cardiomyopathy with Subclinical Heart Failure

Hazel Contractor, Kamaldeep Singh and Ernst von Schwarz

Abstract

Cardiomyopathies consist of a group of cardiac diseases which involve a variety of pathologic entities that result in impaired myocardial cellular activities with subsequent reduced contractile function, oftentimes leading to chronic heart failure. Many patients demonstrate symptoms of heart failure, whereas a subset of patients is relatively asymptomatic without overt signs or symptoms of (congestive) heart failure. Cardiomyopathy with subclinical heart failure is a growing entity that places patients at risk and eventual progression to symptomatologic heart failure. The condition is challenging and nearly impossible to diagnose thus prompts a multi-faceted approach with mindfulness of the cardiac cycle and left ventricular physiology/pathophysiology. This asymptomatic etiology can be uncovered with the assistance of biomarkers, genetic testing, electrocardiogram, echocardiography, X-ray imaging, computer tomography, nuclear scanning, and magnet resonance imaging. Understanding the intricacies of cardiac physiology and pathophysiology while recognizing the limitations of just measuring and relying on ejection fraction may be helpful to risk-stratify individuals earlier to possibly prevent or at least, to delay the progression to overt clinical heart failure and subsequent cardiac death. The lack of a unified dogma for the diagnosis and treatment places a challenge in front of providers and burdens the health care system.

Keywords: cardiomyopathy, heart failure, clinical symptoms, low ejection fraction, hemodynamics

1. Introduction

Cardiomyopathy is characterized as a disease condition that affects the structural and functional abilities of the myocardium. Cardiomyopathies encompass a wide variety of myocardial disorders commonly classified into primary (genetic, non-genetic, or acquired) and secondary cardiomyopathy, which vary in phenotype [1]. According to the American Heart Association, primary cardiomyopathy is defined as a disorder that commonly affects the myocardium itself, whereas secondary cardiomyopathy is a pathologic cardiac involvement as a result of a generalized systemic condition [1]. As this is a generalized classification the most common types of cardiomyopathy present with an underlying pathology of ischemic or non-ischemic origin (**Tables 1** and **2**).

Primary cardiomyopathies
Acquired
Myocarditis
Peripartum
Tachycardia induced
Takotsubo (stress induced)
Genetic
Arrhythmogenic
Hypertrophic
Ion channel disorder
Left ventricular compaction
Mitochondrial myopathies
Mixed
Dilated
Restrictive

Modified from Ref. [1].

Table 1.
Primary cardiomyopathies.

Secondary cardiomyopathies	
Autoimmune	**Infiltrative**
Dermatomyositis	Amyloidosis
Polyarteritis nodosa	Gaucher
Rheumatoid arthritis	Hunter/Hurler syndrome
Sarcoidosis	**Neuromuscular & storage disorders**
Scleroderma	Glycogen storage disorders
SLE	Muscular dystrophy
Endocrine	Neurofibromatosis
Diabetes mellitus	Muscular dystrophy
Thyroid disorders	Neurofibromatosis
Obesity	**Nutritional deficiencies**
Acromegaly	Kwashiorkor
Infectious	Vitamin deficiencies
Chaga's disease	**Toxic**
Hepatitis C	Alcohol
HIV	Chemotherapeutic agents
Rickettsia	Chloroquine
Viral (EBV, Coxsackie, parvo)	Heavy metals
	Hemochromatosis
	Radiation Stimulants

Information from Ref. [1].

Table 2.
Secondary cardiomyopathies.

As cardiomyopathy advances, it triggers myocardial remodeling leading to hypertrophy or loss of contractile materials, interstitial and replacement fibrosis, as well as ventricular and atrial dilatation [1]. These structural modifications cause an inability of the ventricles to efficiently contract or relax, resulting in impaired systolic and diastolic function as known as heart failure.

Consequently, a gradual decline in myocardial function instigates a cascade of hemodynamic abnormalities and neurohormonal activation [2]. Impaired tissue perfusion, elevated filling pressures, and diminished cardiac output collectively

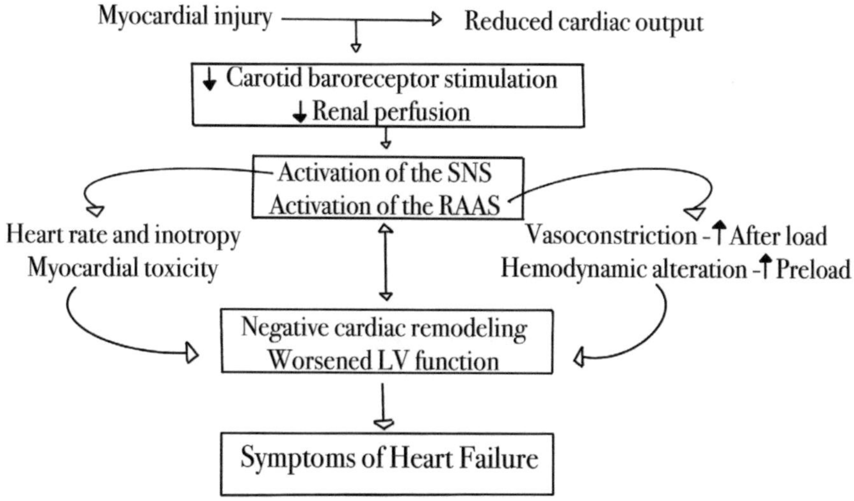

Figure 1.
Heart failure pathophysiology (LV = left ventricle, SNS = sympathetic nervous system, RAAS = renin-angiotensin-aldosterone system).

culminate in the clinical syndrome of heart failure. Neurohormonal activation of the renin-angiotensin-aldosterone system and sympathetic nervous system add to the cycle of myocardial dysfunction and heart failure [2].

Unfortunatley, there is no gold standard diagnostic test for heart failure, therefore, it requires a clinical diagnosis based on history, physical examination, and certain diagnostic testing. Most common causes of heart failure include coronary artery disease, hypertension, idiopathic cardiomyopathy, valvular heart disease, and less commonly, a plethora of different pathologic conditions [3]. Heart failure exhibits a spectrum of signs and symptoms reflective of myocardial dysfunction. Diagnosis of heart failure is verified through a clinical evaluation with positive signs of elevated jugular venous pressure, pulmonary congestion and symptoms of dyspnea, orthopnea, and water accumulation as in edema (lower limb swelling) or pleural effusions or ascites [4]. Symptoms may vary depending on the type of heart failure. On the contrary, identifying cardiomyopathy requires imaging techniques specifying in evaluation of cardiac anatomy, chamber dimensions, morphology, diastolic and systolic function, and valvular pathologies [5]. By classifying cardiomyopathy into ischemic and non-ischemic types, it allows providers to better understand the underlying pathology, proceed with accurate diagnostic evaluations and tailor therapeutic investigations (**Figure 1**).

2. Non-ischemic cardiomyopathy

Non-ischemic cardiomyopathy refers to myocardial diseases that exclude coronary artery disease leading to ischemic insult. These most commonly include hypertrophic cardiomyopathy (HCM), dilated cardiomyopathy (DCM), restrictive cardiomyopathy (RCM), and arrhythmogenic right ventricular cardiomyopathy (ARVCM) [6].

i. Hypertrophic cardiomyopathy (HCM) is an autosomal dominant genetic disease carrying a pathogenic mutation in the cardiac sarcomeric proteins [7]. Most mutations are found in genes encoding beta-myosin heavy chain (MYH7), cardiac myosin binding protein (MYBPC3), or cardiac troponin T (TNNT2) [7]. HCM is characterized by left ventricular hypertrophy with myocyte hypertrophy, disarray, and fibrosis [8]. HCM classically involves the thickening of the basal anterior septal wall, obliterating the left ventricular outflow tract, and mitral regurgitation [8]. Due to these cardiac aberrations, HCM can present with a constellation of symptoms including dyspnea, fatigue palpitations, syncope, chest pain, and sudden cardiac death (SCD) resulting from ventricular arrhythmia [8]. HCM is the most common cause of sudden cardiac death in young adults, therefore risk stratification for SCD relies on prior history of cardiac arrest, family history of sudden death caused by HCM in one or more first degree relative, documentation of a maximum LV wall thickness > 30 mm, and abnormal blood pressure response during exercise [8]. Beyond personal history, physical exam and family history, diagnostic testing involves ECG, non-stress/stress echocardiography and cardiac magnetic resonance [8]. Patients with symptomatic HCM are offered beta-blockers or non-dihydropyridine calcium channel blockers. These medications share their negative inotropic effects resulting in a decrease of systolic anterior motion and left ventricular outflow obstruction [9]. Other medications in use are disopyramide, which reduces the left ventricular outflow gradient and improves survival, angiotensin II receptor blockers, and Mavacamten (Camzyos®), a novel direct myosin inhibitor [10]. Interventional therapies include catheter-based transcutaneous coronary septal ablation and rarely, surgical septal myectomy to mechanically reduce myocardial outflow obstruction [9].

ii. Dilated cardiomyopathy (DCM) is defined by left ventricular or biventricular dilation alongside systolic dysfunction, characterized by abnormal ventricular ejection fraction [11]. DCM can originate from a genetic predisposition or classified as idiopathic if there is no clear genetic link identified. Genetic mutations most commonly occur in the TTN gene encoding the sarcomeric protein, titin. Titin helps to anchor the beta-myosin heavy chains to the Z discs contributing to passive myocardial tension [12]. The phenotype of ventricular dilatation and abnormal contractile dysfunction can be a result of a variety of pathological conditions such as toxins, infections, or autoimmune disorders. Echocardiography is the first line imaging test in providing a diagnosis. Diagnostic echo findings are usually a left ventricular ejection fraction (EF) of less than 45%, normal LV wall thickness, diffuse hypokinesis, right ventricular dilation and dysfunction, and mitral valve and tricuspid valvular regurgitation [13]. Proven pharmacologic therapies include the use of beta blockers, aldosterone antagonists, cardiac glycosides, diuretics, antiarrhythmics, vasodilators, human B-type natriuretic peptides, inotropic agents, and anticoagulation in certain cases. Invasive modalities include valvular repair (or transcutaneous replacement), electric therapy including defibrillator implantations, cardiac resynchronization therapy, the surgical implantation of left ventricular or biventricular mechanical circulatory assist devices, or as the last resort, orthotopic cardiac transplantation [14].

iii. Restrictive cardiomyopathy (RCM) is characterized by diastolic dysfunction of a stiff non-dilated ventricle [15]. There are several causes of RCM, most common are infiltrative pathologies, storage diseases, and a variety of systemic diseases [15]. RCM due to infiltration of abnormal substances between myocytes include diseases such as amyloidosis [15]. Abnormal infiltration of substances within myocytes include hemochromatosis and glycogen storage diseases [15]. Fibrotic injury due to radiation, scleroderma and drugs such as hydroxychloroquine and ergotamine often cause RCM [15]. Echocardiography is the most essential tool when diagnosing patients with RCM. Findings include normal systolic function, bi-atrial enlargement, and abnormal diastolic function [16]. Left ventricular thickness can be normal or increased in patients with infiltrative diseases [16]. Cardiac magnetic resonance imaging can play a crucial role when differentiating constrictive pericarditis from RCM [16]. When non-invasive diagnostics remain equivocal, right ventricular endomyocardial biopsies can be helpful in identifying the underlying pathology [16]. Management involves treating the underlying condition and providing symptomatic therapy for systemic and pulmonary congestion as well as early initiation of heart failure therapies [16].

3. Ischemic cardiomyopathy

For clinical relevance, the first distinction between different forms of cardiomyopathy is between ischemic and non-ischemic cardiomyopathy.

Ischemic cardiomyopathy (ICM) describes a state of left ventricular systolic dysfunction due to past or recurrent or chronic myocardial ischemia [17]. Ischemia is most commonly caused by coronary artery disease (CAD) with or without prior myocardial infarction. ICM is associated with numerous modifiable risks such as diabetes, hypertension, tobacco use, hyperlipidemia, and obesity, and non-modifiable risk factors such as age, gender, and family predisposition [17]. Initially, CAD leads to reduced perfusion of the myocardium, causing reversible loss of cardiac contractile function. If there is a continuous decrease in circulation and oxygenation, irreversible damage to the myocardium results in cardiac cell death, replacement fibrosis, loss of contractile elements, scar formation, ventricular remodeling, and chamber enlargement [18]. Acute or chronic myocardial ischemia might occur as a result of severe coronary artery stenoses due to CAD. This might lead to acute coronary syndromes such as unstable angina, non-ST-segment elevation myocardial infarctions and/or ST-segment elevation myocardial infarctions, characterized by elevated cardiac biomarkers as a result of the presence of necrosis of myocardial cells [18]. Diagnosis of ICM heavily depends on the history and physical examination, EKG, echocardiography and laboratory testing confirm the clinical suspicion.

The following tests are recommended to confirm the diagnosis of ICM:

i. Electrocardiography to detect: ST-segment elevation/ST-segment depression, upright T-wave (STEMI), inverted T-wave (NSTEMI), pathological-Q waves, LBBB [18].

ii. Laboratory test, especially cardiac biomarkers such as cardiac troponins and brain natriuretic peptides (BNP > 35 pg/ml), NT-proBNP >125 pg/ml) [18].

iii. Coronary computed tomographic angiography allows for visualization of the coronary arteries, plaque composition, severity of stenosis, and segments involved [19].

iv. Cardiac imaging such as fractional flow reserve CT might be helpful to measure the ratio between pressures proximal to distal to a stenosis [19].

v. Transthoracic echocardiogram can evaluate left ventricular ejection fraction, left ventricular dysfunction, regional or diffuse wall motion abnormalities, as well as valvular involvement such as mitral and tricuspid regurgitation [18].

vi. Cardiac magnetic resonance: monitoring changes in the left ventricular kinetics after dobutamine administration or by monitoring perfusion under stress with vasodilator drug administration. Late gadolinium enhancement must be used to differentiate perfusion defects caused by ischemia or fibrosis [19].

vii. Stress echocardiography: normokinetic regional wall function at rest and hypokinesia, akinesia or dyskinesia at stress brought upon by exercise or drug administration [19].

viii. Nuclear medicine: myocardial scintigraphy, positron emission tomography (PET); assess the contractile function and regional myocardial blood flow through perfusion tracers and imaging, and single photon emission computed tomography (SPECT); utilizes a radio tracer to evaluate the distribution of blood flow and cell membrane/mitochondrial integrity of the myocardium during stress and at rest [19].

ix. The gold standard for the assessment of the coronary arteries is invasive cardiac catheterization, i.e., coronary angiography to directly visualize the coronary arteries and possibly measure blood flow [19].

Medical management of ischemic cardiomyopathy requires a multifaceted approach in order to improve survival and symptom control.

i. For mortality reduction the following drugs are in use: beta-adrenergic blocking agents, angiotensin-converting enzyme inhibitors or angiotensin II receptor blockers, mineralocorticoid receptor antagonists, and angiotensin receptor neprilysn inhibitors [20].

ii. Symptom management is performed using diuretics, digoxin, ivabradine, and dietary modification [20].

iii. Management of comorbidities such obesity, diabetes, hypertension and sleep disorder are as important as tobacco cessation, and the use of antiplatelet and antithrombotic agents, and lipid-lowering drugs [20].

iv. In case of recurrent ischemia, surgical treatment options might be considered for coronary revascularization using interventional means such as balloon angioplasties with stents or coronary artery bypass surgery, or cardiac transplantation.

4. Cardiomyopathy with HFpEF, HFmrEF, and HFrEF

Initially, cardiomyopathy encompasses structural and functional abnormalities triggering maladaptive myocardial remodeling and compromising the heart's ability to effectively meet the body's metabolic demands. Cardiomyopathy with subclinical heart failure is a common outcome affecting those who have longstanding cardiomyopathy and can be classified according to their diagnostic findings such as ejection fraction. We here distinguish between the two following entities: (1) heart failure with preserved ejection fraction (HFpEF), and (2) heart failure with reduced ejection fraction (HFrEF).

Most commonly, with progressive overload, restrictive and hypertrophic cardiomyopathy tend to evolve into HFpEF due to the diastolic dysfunction while maintaining systolic contraction [21]. High diastolic pressures leading to reduced lung compliance and cardiac output can cause the common signs and symptoms seen in heart failure [21]. Diagnosing heart failure heavily relies on the clinical evidence presented, differentiating between preserved and reduced ejection fraction requires one to seek out further diagnostic measures, which is primary achieved via transthoracic 2-dimensional echocardiography [21]. The HFA-PEFF algorithm for diagnosis of HFpEF was created to provide a clear approach in identifying the problem.

HFpEF on transthoracic echocardiography is characterized by a left ejection fraction of >50% with a non-dilated LV with a normal EF, concentric remodeling or left ventricular hypertrophy, and left atrial enlargement [22]. A comprehensive study is done to measure the mitral early diastolic velocity, left ventricle filling pressure, left atrial volume index, left ventricle mass index, left ventricle wall thickness, tricuspid regurgitation velocity, left ventricle global longitudinal systolic strain, in addition to measure serum natriuretic peptide levels [22]. A score is then developed and grouped into major (2 points) or minor (1 point) criteria. A score of >5 indicates HFpEF, 2–4 indicate diagnostic uncertainty which must move onto step 3, and <1 which HFpEF is unlikely [22]. Treatment for HFpEF must be customized according to patient, however, generally include lifestyle interventions, diuretics, angiotensin receptor-neprilysin inhibitors, angiotensin receptor blockers, mineralocorticoid antagonists, beta blockers, and non-dihydropyridine calcium channel blockers [23].

A third category can be introduced for an ejection fraction of 40–49%, Heart failure with mid-range ejection fraction (HFmrEF) [24]. HFmrEF is an intermediate type of heart failure between HFrEF and HFpEF, although milder, similar characteristics are seen with HFrEF [24]. HFmrEF and HFrEF both share several characteristics such as, ischemic etiology, male sex, younger age, and lower prevalence of atrial fibrillation [24]. HFmrEF patients present with less symptoms and fewer co-morbidities than HFpEF/HFrEF. A possible explanation of the presentation could be due to partially recovered or improved HFrEF patients or worsening HFpEF. When comparing biomarkers, HFmrEF had similar predictors such as levels of NT-pro BNP to HFpEF [25]. Therapeutic evaluations are similar to HFrEF treatment, such as angiotensin-converting enzyme inhibitors, angiotensin-receptor antagonists and β-blockers provide benefit in patients with HFmrEF [25]. Since the establishment of HFmrEF, the knowledge for this subtype continues to evolve and with newer findings allowing a better understanding of the clinical profile.

Heart failure with reduced left ventricular ejection fraction (HFrEF) is defined as a reduced ejection fraction of <40%, also described as *systolic* heart failure [26]. HFrEF is characterized by eccentric remodeling accompanied with ventricular dilatation and volume overload [27]. HFrEF is observed more often in patients with coronary artery disease and previous myocardial infarction [27]. Dilated and ischemic cardiomyopathy both are accompanied by systolic dysfunction triggering the development of HFrEF. Pharmacologic therapy for HFrEF can include a combination of diuretics, ARBs/ACEi/ARNIs, hydralazine plus nitrate, beta-blockers, mineralocorticoid receptor antagonists, digoxin, ivabradine, and sodium glucose cotransport 2 inhibitors [28]. In the case where pharmacologic therapies are not improving the symptoms, additional therapies with cardiac implantable devices have shown to be beneficial to improve mortality and reduce the chance of sudden cardiac death [28].

Patients with HFrEF/HFpEF can experience signs and symptoms of heart failure through many compensatory mechanisms which may overwhelm the entire organism. In the initial stages of heart failure, the increased wall stress leads to myocyte hypertrophy, cell death, and some compensation [29]. Continuous myocardial insult causes eccentric remodeling, further worsening the stress on the remaining myocytes, resulting in decreased cardiac output. A decrease in cardiac output can clinically as fatigue, weakness, and decreased exercise tolerance [29]. Maladaptive myocardial changes activate hemodynamic and neurohormonal derangements that further exacerbate signs and symptoms of clinically manifest heart failure. Activation of the sympathetic system leads to the release of epinephrine and norepinephrine causing vasoconstriction, which increases both calcium afterload and entry of cytosolic calcium [29]. These changes augment myocardial contractility and relaxation, at least for a while. At the same time, afterload might increase as well as the incidence of ventricular arrhythmia. Increased afterload caused by vasoconstriction further contributes to shortness of breath and fatigue [29]. In addition, activation of the RAAS leads to increased levels of angiotensin II, in turn, increased aldosterone levels, which also support sodium and water retention, leading to pulmonary congestion, dyspnea, peripheral edema, gastro-intestinal congestion, and ascites [29].

A majority of HFpEF/HFrEF patients present with heart failure symptoms, thus allowing further investigation to diagnose and manage accordingly. When HFpEF/HFrEF patients are *asymptomatic*—meaning there are no overt symptoms of any condition including cardiovascular pathologies evident, the diagnosis rather is established incidentally upon routine non symptom related evaluations. Since the cardiac pathology is neither expected nor verified, outcome become more unpredictable and dangerous as there is a lack or delay of sufficient medical management with subsequently increased mortality. A large proportion of asymptomatic patients with newly diagnosed cardiomyopathy with heart failure live sedentary lifestyles and therefore, might not feel or report any of the classical HF symptoms under usual resting conditions [30, 31]. Also, younger individuals may have less co-morbidities such obesity, hypertension and diabetes, and possess a higher cardiac reserve, allowing them to be more tolerant towards initial myocardial damage without experiencing symptoms [30, 31]. Patients might also learn to adapt to the condition through lifestyle changes [30, 31]. Neurohormonal activation of the SNS and RAAS are able to temporarily maintain a sufficient cardiac output and adequate tissue perfusion, thus delaying the onset of any heart failure symptoms [32]. Early detection, diagnosis, and initiation of effective medical management can play a pivotal role in asymptomatic heart failure in order to delay the progression of the disease and to avoid early death.

Symptoms in patients with HFr/EF and with HFpEF are commonly very similar—regardless of ejection fraction. HFpEF has similar pathophysiologic processes as HFrEF, with HFpEF responding to increased ventricular stiffness and altered relaxation, and HFrEF responding to cardiac output [28]. Both conditions lead to activation of the sympathetic nervous system and renin angiotensin activating system causing an increase in heart rate, vasoconstriction, and fluid retention. HFrEF and HFpEF contribute to increased afterload through different mechanisms [28]. HFrEF increases afterload through systemic vasoconstriction and hypertension, whereas HFpEF increases afterload through increased pulmonary vascular resistance [28]. These compensatory mechanisms cause further stress to the heart, worsening ventricular function, and leading to similar symptoms. Abnormalities in left ventricular filling pressures better correlate to occurrence and severity of symptoms compared to left ventricular ejection fraction (**Table 3**).

HSA-PEFF algorithm for the diagnosis of HFpEF	
Initial workup (Step 1 (P): Pretest Assessment)	• Symptoms/signs of HF • Co-morbidities/Risk factors • ECG • Standard Echocardiography • Natriuretic peptides • Ergometry/6 min walking test or cardiopulmonary exercise testing
Diagnostic workup (Step 2 (E): echocardiographic and natriuretic peptide score)	• Comprehensive echocardiography • Natriuretic peptides, if not measured in step 1
Advanced workup (Step 3 (F1): functional testing in case of uncertainty)	• Diastolic stress test: exercise stress echocardiography • Invasive hemodynamic measurements
Etiological workup (Step 4 (F2): final etiology)	• Cardiovascular magnetic resonance • Cardiac or non cardiac biopsies • Scintigraphy/CT/PET • Genetic testing • Specific laboratory tests

HFA-PEFF = heart failure association pre test assessment, echocardiography and natriuretic peptide score.
Modified from Ref. [20].

Table 3.
HFpEF.

5. Cardiomyopathy with reduced cardiac output

Heart failure is a common debilitating illness, and it is associated with significant morbidity and mortality, frequent hospitalization, and enormous psychological and socioeconomic burdens. Current guidelines almost invariably emphasize the management of patients with symptomatic disease. However, patients invariably have a period when the left ventricular function is decreased or is decreasing but have minimal to no symptoms. Ideally, one would like to identify these individuals before symptoms develop, but this may be difficult or in many cases, impossible.

As providers delineate heart failure patients into groups, these are based on ejection fraction, systolic or diastolic heart failure, acute, chronic, or acute on chronic heart failure, New York Heart Association (NYHA) functional classification (I-IV), and the American Heart Association/American College of Cardiology (ACC/AHA) staging (A–D). While this may provide a phenotype for a patient to assign a trajectory for prognosis and treatment, this may leave patients with subclinical heart failure cardiomyopathy untreated and at-risk. These patients require health care providers to look at many factors beyond these and to consider the overall function of the heart as a pump within the clinical picture. In this frame, the challenge then arises regarding an asymptomatic cardiomyopathic patient with reduced or preserved cardiac output. This brings to question what a provider must anticipate to preventing the progression to clinically overt heart failure. One might classify such patients in stage B heart failure (asymptomatic but with structural changes), and then, initiate appropriate management to reduce disease progression and adverse outcomes [33]. Clearly, the earlier patients with heart failure are identified—independent on symptomatology—the better the prognosis will be.

Asymptomatic left ventricular systolic dysfunction is classified as stage B heart failure according to the AHA/ACC guidelines [33]. It is defined as decreased left ventricular systolic function in the absence of clinical symptoms. Early initiation of therapies in patients with presumed asymptomatic left ventricular systolic dysfunction (ALVSD) has been shown to lead to improve eventual outcomes [34]. ALVSD has been found to be in a similar distribution amongst the population as symptomatic congestive HF [35].

Understanding EF and the challenges that arise when attempting to classify cardiomyopathy with low cardiac output as a homogenous syndrome can test a provider's understanding to the limitations of EF itself. The definition of EF, in 1962 by Folse and Braunwald, was described as fraction of left ventricular volume ejected per beat [36]. EF is an interpretation of instantaneous change in ventricular ejection where the stroke volume (SV) is expressed as an a instantaneous portion of end-diastolic volume (EDV). This provides data as a measure of change in contractility under stable load conditions. Changes of the myocardial cell structure may predispose to an increase or decrease in LVEDV and influence the EF at a given level of contractility and SV. A provider must keep in mind that EF is influenced by both preload (diastole) and afterload (systole), and interpreting EF as an index of contractility without knowledge of left ventricular (LV) loads may lead to unnecessary intervention.

Pressure-volume curves best demonstrate the disengagement of EF from contractility. In a normal heart, the preload increase is demonstrated as an increase in EDV, increased SV & contractile force by the Frank-Starling mechanism [37]. An increase in vascular resistance is demonstrated by afterload, increased arterial pressure and contractile force, maintaining SV & increasing stroke work [37]. This results in minimal changes, increases contractile force, maintains cardiac output, and an unchanged EF [38].

Cardiac remodeling in HF results in a decrease in myocardial contractility as well as SV and EF. The decrease in stroke volume can be observed by the simultaneous decrease in cardiac output. In DCM, EF may be lower due to a larger EDV [39] as compared to that of HCM. Cardiac remodeling and reduced cavitary volume result in an increased EF instead of an increased SV or contractility in HCM.

LVEF as a measure of LV function has important limitations to consider, such as technical limitations affecting the calculated EF. Left ventricular ejection fraction is an indirect measurement by imaging techniques, such as echocardiography, where an EF is calculated from an estimate volume of the LV [40]. Clear technical challenges include inferior image quality, challenging anatomy that leads to foreshortened ventricles, delineation of the endocardium with boundary continuity that may be out of view, inter/intra-observer variability, and semi-automatic delineation applications with similar issues without standardization and questionable reproducibility [40]. Data shows repeat measures of ejection fraction in an individual over a period of time can result in a 5- to 7-point variability [41]. It is essential to remember that LVEF is calculated as a volume-derived index, requires geometric assumptions (using one/two-dimensional echocardiography), and is heavily load-dependent.

Prior studies instituted different definitions for impaired LVEF, usually <50% to the less common <35%. This creates a range of individuals with different phenotypes with the risk of progression and prognosis without symptoms. Clearly, decreases in LVEF correspond with eventual outcomes [42, 43] and an inverse relationship between LVEF and mortality reaches a steady state near a LVEF of 40–45%, above which LVEF may not correspond to mortality [43]. As a facet of ventricular function,

EF creates division of systole and diastole, rather than evaluation of cardiac function through the cardiac cycle. This may result in an exclusion of the possible role of diastolic function and its prognostic value [44, 45].

As mentioned earlier, LVEF is influenced by loading conditions of the LV, and thus is not a true surrogate for intrinsic myocardial contractility [40]. LVEF can remain normal in lieu of LV dysfunction, i.e., LV hypertrophy and/or decreased cavity size, leading to a decreased stroke volume [46]. Clearly, a rationale limited by LVEF may omit ventricular function in the cardiac cycle.

A reliance on EF may prompt a provider to use an inotrope that can improve symptomatology in the acute phase yet worsen the underlying pathology and increase mortality [47]. The geometry of the LV can influence the LVEF, for example in athletes with an enlarged LV cavity marginally lower LVEF values may be observed, [41] increased LVEF is often observed in various forms of LV hypertrophy, [48] and in ventricular dys-synchrony such as left bundle branch block. In this scenario, the largest LV volume may not reflect the end-diastolic volume and interfere with the performed LVEF measurement. Tachycardia also impacts LVEF as will be decreased in this state and in states where cardiac contractility is increased, i.e., use of dobutamine [40].

The pattern of contraction of the ventricle should be considered as HF evolves, separate from global/regional systolic function. Strain measurements may provide meaningful contractility data as a change in EF can mark ventricular remodeling rather than a distinction in contractility. In systole, the shortening of longitudinal fibers causes the movement of the LV basal plane towards a relatively anchored apex. Simultaneously, there is a shortening of circumferential fibers which generates an inward deformation towards the LV cavity of the LV myocardium (radial thickening). Since the deformation in both planes will reduce LV volume in systole, using LVEF will correspond to the function of both longitudinal/circumferential LV fibers thus lacking the dexterity to characterize a defect of one of the components. Incapacitation or impairment of longitudinal function can happen prior to the same in circumferential function, presenting as a subclinical impairment of LV pump function. Circumferential function, to an extent, compensates for the commencing decrease in longitudinal function. In a hypertrophied heart, LVEF and fractional shortening are both above normal while longitudinal function may be impaired [48–52]. Strain can also be used to calculate mechanical dispersion, as the standard deviation of the time to peak strain. Mechanical dispersion has been shown to be a predictor of arrhythmias in ischemic and other forms of cardiomyopathies [53].

6. Cardiomyopathy with preserved cardiac output

Asymptomatic left ventricular diastolic dysfunction (ALVDD) is defined by the presence of diastolic dysfunction with a normal EF in the absence of symptoms [54]. Focusing on ischemic HFrEF provides the basis for this definition with decreased LVEF, abnormal regional myocardial contractility, LV enlargement, hypertrophy, or valvular disease. Diagnosing stage B heart failure may be challenging or impossible in non-ischemic etiologies typically delineated as preserved EF, i.e., in patients with obesity, diabetes, and hypertension. Invariably, LV diastolic dysfunction and impaired global longitudinal strain (GLS) may be pragmatic [55–59].

The extended stage B heart failure (SBHF) definition is consistent with the concept of early myocardial disease presented in the 2016 ASE/EACVI guidelines on diastolic function [60]. As both LV diastolic and longitudinal systolic impairment may develop in parallel and may originate from a shared pathological etiology. The presence of impaired global longitudinal strain (GLS) or measures of longitudinal contractility support diastolic dysfunction as they correspond to myocardial impairment, while not always occurring concomitantly. Both LV diastolic and longitudinal systolic impairment contribute to a decrease in exercise capacity [61] possibly preceding the development of symptomatic HF. Diastolic dysfunction should be recognized with synergistic pathologies such as altered LV contractility and myocardial cell structure changes, i.e. LV hypertrophy and remodeling. In addition to contributing to exercise intolerance, these features are associated with progression from stage A through stage B to symptomatic HF [55, 56, 62, 63].

There exists the need to broaden the definition of stage B HF as the known definition relies on LVEF and LV structural criteria [55, 56, 62, 64]. Incorporation of both diastolic function and GLS into a screening echocardiographic protocol may help to identify individuals predisposed to develop HF [64]. Risk prediction for HF may benefit from utilizing LV diastolic and longitudinal deformation parameters as a more broad pathophysiology may be uncovered in the earlier phases of cardiac dysfunction. In HF due to non-ischemic pathology, relying on EF based definitions for stage B HF may omit at-risk cases [65].

Deformation imaging demonstrates the rate of deformation or strain rate and shows correlation with sonomicrometry information, less dependence on load as compared to LVEF, [66, 67] and elucidates myocardial impairment in preserved LVEF [68, 69]. As compared to EF, Doppler-based deformation analysis may take longer to master. Speckle tracking can provide analysis with deformation curves and information that is more palpable to interpretation due to spatial smoothing. A limitation to this technique is the reliance on semi-automatic image segmentation (delineation) and quantification techniques to provide a reproducible platform [40].

EFs limited role in predicting at risk patients with heart failure and preserved LVEF paves the potential role for myocardial deformation imaging in the evaluation of patients with HFpEF. Studies demonstrate impairment of LV longitudinal function in HFpEF [70–74]. Longitudinal strain has been found to be reduced in HFpEF patients with hypertensive cardiomyopathy [50] while circumferential fibers and LVEF were maintained proposing a compensatory mechanism for impaired longitudinal function similar to that of diabetic patients [51, 52]. Notably, diminished circumferential strain in these HFpEF patients was correlated with decreased systolic blood pressure and stroke volume, indicating that impairment of both circumferential fibers and longitudinal fibers may be a mechanism in the development of HFpEF [48, 50, 75]. Individuals with HFpEF have demonstrated a reduction in longitudinal strain and this has been established as the most important echocardiographic predictor of cardiovascular death or HF [76].

7. Management

7.1 Medical therapy

The symptomatology of heart failure results from excessive salt and water retention leading to pathologic volume expansion of the vascular/extravascular spaces. While medical management or device/surgical management is reserved for symptomatic heart failure, the importance of these modalities should not be understated. We briefly describe the mechanism of action and role of these medications.

i. *Loop diuretics* will act on the Na-K2Cl symporter found on the apical membrane of epithelial cells in the thick ascending loop of Henle by competing with chloride's binding site. The resulting loss of up to 2–25% of the filtered load of sodium and free water excretion will affect intracardiac pressure as well as hemodynamic parameters. When administered intravenously, this class of medications act as venous dilators and decrease right atrial pressure as well as pulmonary capillary wedge pressure rapidly possibly from a release of prostaglandins that cause vasodilation. A rise in systemic vascular resistance can also be seen due to temporary activation of renin-angiotensin system by direct stimulation of macula densa cells to secrete renin and ultimately raise LV afterload [77].

ii. *Thiazide diuretics* are known to block the Na-Cl transporter that is found in the cortical segment of the ascending loop of Henle as well as the distal convoluted tubule resulting in an increase of 5–10% of the fractional excretion of the filtered load of sodium. A decrease in free water clearance and loss of potency in individuals with impaired renal function may be observed. Notably, the Na-Cl cotransporter can be found within the vascular space and other types of cells in other organs, possibly enhancing the utility as antihypertensive medications [77]. Thiazide diuretics do not alter mortality in HF patients.

iii. *Aldosterone antagonists* are mild diuretics and used in HF. Aldosterone binds to cytosolic receptors (ligand-dependent transcription factors) in the distal nephron. Then these translocate to the nucleus of the cell followed by binding to hormone response elements present in the promoter area of genes (involved in vascular/myocardial fibrosis, inflammation, & calcification). Synthetic mineralocorticoid receptors, also known as mineralocorticoid receptor antagonists, decrease the activity of the Na-K exchange (where aldosterone has its effect) on the distal nephron. Spironolactone and canrenone (active metabolite), competitively inhibit aldosterone's ability to bind to MRA/type I receptors across tissues such as cells found in the distal convoluted tubules and collecting ducts. This quality to upset the renin-angiotensin aldosterone system provides its utility in treatment for heart failure [77]. Aldosterone antagonists improve mortality in HF.

iv. *Potassium sparing diuretics*, as organic bases, are transported into the proximal tubule followed by blockade of Na reabsorption in the late distal tubule and collecting duct [77].

v. *Carbonic anhydrase inhibitors* can impede zinc metalloenzyme carbonic anhydrase followed by a virtually complete loss of proximal tubular $NaHCO_3$ resorption. Other diuretics may cause a contraction phenomenon resulting in a metabolic alkalosis prompting the temporary use of this class of medication [77].

vi. *Sodium-Glucose Transporter-2 inhibitors* act on the SGLT-2 transporter found in the S1 & S2 segments of the proximal tubule. Not only is the transporter responsible for 90% of the glucose reabsorption the kidneys, it is also responsible for proximal tubular reabsorption of sodium, and absorption of chloride. The resulting contraction of the plasma volume, without activation of the sympathetic nervous system, is accompanied by a modest decrease in blood pressure. The site of action of this class of medication demonstrates a decrease in glomerular filtration by afferent arteriole vasoconstriction through tubule-glomerular feedback [77].

vii. The pituitary hormone AVP, elevated in HF, can increase systemic vascular resistance as well as promote a positive water balance. *Combined V1a/V2 antagonists* result in reduced systemic vascular resistance and can prohibit dilutional hyponatremia in HF. AVP has notable effects based on this receptor subtype. Selective V1a antagonists act by blocking the vasoconstrictive effects and resulting myocardial hypertrophy in vascular smooth muscle. By inhibiting the conscription of aquaporin water channels into the epithelial cell apical membrane of collecting duct, the ability to reabsorb water decreases [77].

viii. Angiotensin converting enzyme inhibitors (ACEIs) inhibit the enzyme that is responsible for the conversion of angiotensin I to angiotensin II. By interfering with the RAS system, this class of medications can stabilize LV myocardial cell structure changes, ameliorate clinical symptoms, reduce hospitalization, and potentially extend life.

ix. *Angiontensin II receptor blockers* (ARBs) inhibit the effect of angiotensin II on the angiotensin type 1 receptor, thus providing the ability to fend off the detrimental effects of angiotensin II on cardiac remodeling [77].

x. New therapeutic class of agents that antagonize RAAS and inhibit the neutral endopeptidase system combines an ARB, valsartan, with *sacubitril* (a *neprilysin inhibitor (NI)*). This combination of an ARB with an NI is abbreviated ARNI and has been shown to reduce the breakdown of natriuretic peptides, bradykinin, and adrenomedullin while inhibiting renin and aldosterone secretion. These effects then promote diuresis, natriuresis, and myocardial relaxation. AT1-receptor blockade additionally decreases vasoconstriction, sodium/water retention, and myocardial hypertrophy [77].

xi. *Beta-adrenergic receptor blockers* are a notable class of medications; a provider will find themselves deciding to start or not start in cardiomyopathy with subclinical heart failure. Their mechanism of action works by competitive inhibition of one or more adrenergic receptors (α1, β1 and β2). The greatest harmful effects of sympathetic activation are mediated by the β1 adrenergic receptor. The functional effects of beta-blocker therapy on the failing heart are biphasic, as an early, transient worsening of cardiac function due to the negative inotropic effects of rescinding adrenergic drive. When given gradually with slow up-titration in relatively euvolemic individuals this deterioration may not be apparent. When administered with ACEIs, a reduction in LV volumes from possible negation of LV remodeling, improved changes in LV contour, and augmented LVEF. Over time when beta-blockers are given with ACEIs, they have been found to ameliorate clinical symptoms and reduce hospitalization while prolonging life [77].

xii. *Ivabradine*, a heart rate-lowering medication, selectively blocks the "funny" (If) cardiac current that controls the spontaneous diastolic depolarization of the sinoatrial node. By acting in a concentration-dependent manner and entering the channel pore from the intracellular side, the channel will be blocked when it is open. Thus the level of If inhibition is directly related to how often the channel opens thus would be effective with higher heart rate states [77].

xiii. In HF, an imbalance exists between oxidative stress and nitric oxide (NO) availability where a reduction in NO bioavailability predisposes to endothelial dysfunction as well as LV dysfunction. *Vericiguat*, a oral soluble *guanylate cyclase stimulator*, magnifies the cyclic guanosine monophosphate (GMP) production pathway by direct stimulation of soluble guanylate cyclase activity and sensitize this to endogenous NO [77].

xiv. *Cardiac myosin activators* increase myocardial contractility without increasing intracellular concentrations of cyclic adenosine mono-phosphate, calcium, and myocardial oxygen consumption. *Omecamtiv mecarbil*, a small-molecule activator of myosin, is found to prolongs myocardial systole by increasing the proportion of sarcomeric myosin molecules that are strongly bound to actin and thus leading to generation of myocardial force and contractility [77].

xv. *Digitalis glycosides* such as *digoxin* and *digitoxin* are the most frequently used cardiac glycosides, especially in chronic HF. Digoxin's inhibits the sodium potassium adenosine trisphosphate (Na-K+ ATPase) pump in cell membranes, including the sarcolemmal NaK+ ATPase pump of cardiac myocytes. This inhibition of Na-K+ ATPase pump promotes an increase in intracellular calcium and resulting increased cardiac contractility. Additionally, in patients with HF digoxin can sensitize Na+K+ ATPase activity in vagal afferent nerves that will stabilize the excess activation of the adrenergic system in advanced HF. Digoxin also inhibits Na-K+ ATPase activity in the kidney and may therefore blunt renal tubular resorption of sodium [77]. Cardiac glycosides are mainly used in HF patients with uncontrolled atrial fibrillation with elevated heart rates.

Inotropic agents such as dobutamine, dopamine, milrinone, adrenaline an d norepinephrine are reserved for intravenous therapy for patients in cardiogenic shock. BNP is also less frequently used for aggressive IV diuresis and afterload reduction, as is nitroprusside sodium. Experimental evidence suggests a role of *n-3 polyunsaturated fatty acids* (PUFA) with reassuring effects on inflammation. These effects include reducing endothelial activation with production of inflammatory cytokines, platelet aggregation, autonomic tone, blood pressure, heart rate, and LV function [77].

7.2 Electrical therapy including cardiac contractility modulation (CCM)

Altered myocardial contractility can lead to HF with a variety of secondary manifestations. These include neurohormonal activation, autonomic imbalance, arrhythmias, ventricular dyssynchrony, myocardial remodeling, secondary mitral regurgitation (SMR), sleep disordered breathing, and sudden cardiac death. While usually reserved for advanced HF, the utility of electrical therapy in this scenario cannot be understated.

Sudden cardiac death may be the first manifestation of ventricular arrhythmia in heart failure, placing importance in the use of prophylactic defibrillator-cardioverter (ICD) implantation to prevent sudden cardiac death (SCD) [78]. ICDs treat the ventricular arrhythmias that still occur despite optimized medical therapy in HFrEF patients. In current practice, defibrillators are utilized in select high-risk patients who have not experienced a prior sudden cardiac arrest event or a sustained ventricular arrythmia, usually those with a maintained EF of equal or less than 35%. Interestingly, a large number of individuals that receive defibrillators do not develop life-threatening ventricular arrhythmia that would require anti-tachycardia intervention. This places an importance on the need to further improve risk prediction/stratification [79] beyond LVEF by noninvasive means including clinical, imaging, electrophysiological, genetic, and biological markers. Examples include signal-averaged ECG, reduced heart rate variability, T wave or repolarization changes, and myocardial scarring on late gadolinium enhancement by magnetic resonance imaging.

Intraventricular conduction abnormalities are associated with increased morbidity and mortality in chronic HF [80]. Electrical dysynchrony, defined as a QRS duration greater than 120 msec on the ECG, results from a difference in the timing of mechanical contraction or relaxation between different segments of the LV with resulting in inefficient ventricular filling, decreased in LV contractility, worsened mitral regurgitation (MR), and paradoxical septal wall motion [81]. Roughly one-third of patients with HFrEF have been found to have ventricular dyssynchrony as evidenced by left bundle branch block [81]. Studies have demonstrated the utility of cardiac resynchronization therapy (CRT) in patients with HFrEF and ventricular dyssynchrony on improvement in hemodynamics, functional outcomes, quality of life (QoL), and morbidity/mortality benefits [82]. CRT is provided by using am additional left ventricular electrode in a pacemaker or defibrillator inserted via the coronary vein to stimulate the left ventricle.

CardioMEMS is a heart sensor is an implantable hemodynamic monitor that can be placed into a pulmonary artery with the ability to transmit pulmonary pressures electronically and thus allow a provider to make therapeutic adjustments [83].

Placement of an intra-atrial shunting device between the LA and RA with resulting lower LA pressures at rest states and exertion states. While still experimental, early data has shown the potential for a safe method that may improve hemodynamics [84, 85]. Additionally this technique has been found reduction of pulmonary artery diastolic/systolic pressures, a significant decrease in HF-related events, days alive out of hospital, and improvement in quality of life. Notably, similar findings were observed in patients across varying EFs possibly positioning this technique to improve outcomes in the more challenging to diagnose HF patients such as HFpEF and HFmrEF [84, 85].

Cardiac contractility modulation (CCM) is a newer, innovative device-based therapy in the management of HF. CCM uses multiple electrodes to deliver relatively high-voltage (~7.5 V) biphasic signals to the endocardium of the RV septum with resulting improvement of HF symptomatology, exercise capacity, and quality of life [86–88]. CCM can alter the expression of cytoskeletal proteins and myofilaments with resulting decreased fibrosis and improving contractility [89]. The reverse remodeling observed with CCM appears similar to one induced by CRT in patients with a modestly prolonged QRS [90]. CCM has been shown to improve myocardial contractility without a concomitant increase in myocardial oxygen consumption [91, 92]. Understanding every myocardial segment contributes to cardiac pump function, CCM has the potential for global improvement in myocardial contraction, i.e. regions remote to impulse delivery [93]. Notably, improved physical functioning and reduced hospital admissions were observed using this electrical treatment [94].

Central sleep apnea is a finding in advanced HF. The Remede system (Respicardia, Minnetonka, MN) was FDA approved in 2017 for the treatment of moderate to severe CSA in adult patients. A study with individuals stratified by NYHA Class I-IV, demonstrated a ≥ 50% reduction in Apnea-Hypopnea Index (AHI) from baseline at 6 months [95]. Another study in HFrEF, however, demonstrated no change in primary endpoints, time to death from any cause, lifesaving cardiac intervention, or hospitalization for worsening HF symptomatology while showing worse all-cause and cardiovascular mortality [96].

Baroreflex activation therapy (BAT) is designed to restore this autonomic imbalance by inhibiting the sympathetic system and activating the parasympathetic system by electrically stimulating the baroreceptors in the carotid sinus. The BAROSTIM NEO system (CVRx, Inc., Minneapolis, MN), consists of a pulse generator and a carotid sinus lead implanted surgically to deliver BAT [97–99]. This is relevant as HF has been shown to exhibit an autonomic imbalance with enhanced activity of the sympathetic nervous system concomitant decreased parasympathetic activation. The resulting increased heart rate, blood pressures, myocardial cell structure changes, decreased diuresis, and elevated renin secretion all portend an increase in morbidity/mortality.

7.3 Surgical therapies

While the focus of symptomatic HF treatment is medical or electrical, some patients may require invasive/surgical intervention. We briefly discuss current guideline recommended surgical options.

7.3.1 PCI/coronary artery bypass grafting

Coronary artery disease (CAD) is the most common cause of HF by mechanisms of acute/chronic ischemia as well as myocardial infarction (MI) [100]. Repetitive myocardial ischemic insult results in myocardial hibernation that leads to reduced LV function followed by clinically overt HF. Revascularization, by coronary artery bypass grafting (CABG), provides the basis to reversing this hibernation of myocardium in CAD and HF. This treatment has shown to improve survival in patients with HFrEF [101]. Obstructive epicardial CAD is likely under-recognized in patients with HFpEF given epicardial CAD is commonly seen with HFpEF with evidence of obstructive CAD in nearly half of patients with HFpEF [102–104]. Revascularization with PCI may also be useful and beneficial in these scenarios, especially if extensive solutions are in sight, and holds the benefit of less procedural hazard of CABG in these individuals with HF.

7.3.2 Valve repair/replacement

Valvular disease that is not rectified, such as mitral regurgitation (MR), may result in diastolic HF. The change in LV cell structure, caused by ischemic or dilated cardiomyopathy, is observed by displacement of papillary muscles and tethering of leaflets that ultimately causes MR [105, 106]. MR further will worsen LV function with corresponding adverse clinical outcomes from the progression LV cell structure change [105]. The presence of both MR and HF worsens prognosis of these patients and this makes MR a therapeutic target [107]. Surgery is not recommended in patients with severe MR where the risk may be high. In these patients guideline-directed medical therapy and transcatheter edge-to-edge repair (TEER) may be recommended [108]. MitraClip, commonly used device of TEER, has been shown to be safer than surgery, improve NYHA functional class, and overall survival [109, 110].

7.3.3 Heart transplantation

In advanced HF, when optimal medical therapy, as recommended by the ACC/AHA guidelines, and cardiac resynchronization therapy have not successfully improved symptoms or deterred progression of disease in advanced HF, heart transplant may be considered [111–114]. The indications for this procedure are well studied and include nonischemic cardiomyopathy, ischemic cardiomyopathy, valvular heart disease, re-transplantation, and others [115–117].

8. Future directions in the epidemiology, diagnosis and management of cardiomyopathy with subclinical heart failure

As the ratio of individuals with obesity, diabetes, and hypertension grows so does the prevalence of cardiomyopathy with subclinical heart failure. This may potentially be mitigated by the routine screening for HF with biomarkers/imaging, however, there is a lack of a payments for this in spite of the benefits, i.e., decreased costs of health care as well as better outcomes. A viable strategy would be to implement this into the current guidelines and standards to nudge insurers to pay for this. Screening may be a powerful asset to a provider working with populations of greater concern including obesity, diabetes, hypertension, coronary artery disease, cardiotoxicity, or a genetic history of cardiomyopathy. Utilizing genetic testing, cardiac troponins, natriuretic peptides, electrocardiogram, echocardiogram, and cardiac MRI will facilitate a provider in the assessment of true cardiac function and cell structure.

Upon the recognition of cardiomyopathy in subclinical heart failure, there are methods by which a patient may take an advantage of early diagnosis in the asymptomatic phase. Early, thorough education of a patient will equip them with this through abstinence from tobacco products, unrestricted alcohol use, participation in consistent exercise, eating heart-healthy diet, and control of glucose levels, cholesterol levels, and blood pressure. A patient such as this may benefit from the accessibility of digital apps, routine follow up, and support groups. The public health sector should be motivated to elevate general public awareness regarding healthy lifestyle changes as well as the role for screening, and treatment of this disease. Invariably, a unified dogma that incorporates the many facets of the health sector (general public, insurers, health care organizations, providers, and makers of policy) will be necessary to mitigate the increasing prevalence of the disease.

In earlier sections we have detailed medical, electrical, & surgical treatment options. Treatment should target the maintenance of therapy to optimize obesity, diabetes, hypertension, ischemic cardiac disease, and valvular cardiac pathology. Employing a multi-disciplinary approach may be useful in these patients as well as those exposed to cardiotoxicity. ACE/ARBs, SGLT2 inhibitors, and beta blockers have been well studied and benefits of these medications include preventing the progression of cardiomyopathy with subclinical HF to a symptomatic phenotype and a reduction of mortality. At present, there is a paucity of evidence for a recommendation of ARNIs in asymptomatic LV dysfunction or cardiomyopathy with subclinical heart failure. The recommendation for SGLT2 inhibitors may arise in the near future once studies examine this medication's effects in patients having myocardial infarction with or without LV dysfunction or HF.

9. Clinical scenarios and unresolved issues

Various scenarios may prompt a provider to elucidate asymptomatic patients, for example in the clinic, during an annual exam (or an insurance exam) with an abnormal family history (especially of younger relatives), ECG, or a murmur may warrant further workup. Additionally, often times screening vehicles/camps in the community may report similar findings. Some patients may report shortness of breath at high altitudes more so than others. In the hospital, when patients are admitted with a different non-cardiovascular illness (i.e. pneumonia, gastrointestinal bleed) can have a non-specific ECG with an abnormal echo followed by initiation of a beta blocker therapy inpatient, and post-hospitalization recovery with normalized cardiac function on follow up. When pacing from the RV, a HF patient may still be symptomatic with a normal LVEF denoting abnormality of the method of conduction and warranting a pacemaker revision. Obstructive sleep apnea may be another source as initially there may be asymptomatic LV dysfunction.

Heart failure is a clinical diagnosis, whereas cardiomyopathy is usually established by a form of imaging. Early onset HFrEF may be asymptomatic as the underlying asymptomatic ventricular systolic dysfunction has yet to progress to overt, symptomatologic HF. Likewise, with HFpEF, early in the course of the disease a patient may be without symptoms and later may also progress from asymptomatic left ventricular diastolic dysfunction to over, symptomatic HF. During this early period individuals that have cardiomyopathy with subclinical heart failure are challenging to identify, treat, and label as "heart failure." Once the underlying progresses, both HFrEF and HFpEF may manifest similarly as left ventricular function becomes compromised and results in decreased cardiac output. Cardiomyopathy with low EF can have low cardiac output and manifest with clinical symptoms. Cardiomyopathy with low EF may also have a preserved, maintained and normal cardiac output while asymptomatic due to preserved EDV/preload, contractility/deformation, and SVR/afterload. This is important when dealing with early myocardial disease where the strain may be abnormal first, as seen in hypertensive, obese, or diabetic patients. This concept underpins the importance of understanding ventricular physiology, pathology, and echocardiography findings such as GLS and measuring true cardiac output.

The pathophysiology of HF, regardless of LVEF, is characterized by insufficient cardiac output. Despite normal or mildly reduced LVEF, stroke volume (cardiac output) can be low in patients with HFpEF and HFrEF because of a proportionate small LV volume and LA failure, resulting in the inability to change stroke volume during exertion relying on elevating filling pressures. Cardiac output may be adequate at rest states and manifest with symptoms during exertion.

In HFrEF, manipulation of stroke volume has potential for treatment in HF. In scenarios with higher LVEF, as in HFpEF, an increase in contractility is questionable as these patients exhibit LV systolic dysfunction with impaired contractility. Chronotropic incompetence may result in HF symptomatology as there is an inability to appropriately increase heart rate in the setting of exertion/exercise, especially in HFpEF & HFmrEF [118].

Several HFpEF phenotypic subtypes may be present due to the varying nature of the HFpEF syndrome, its mechanisms, and endothelial dysfunction affecting multiple organ [119]. This demonstrated why a single, simple, agreed upon classification system has not been out of reach. As a disconnect is present between calculated EF and true cardiac output, the criterion used for classification with NYHA, class, staging for differentiation of heart failure are insufficient. Recognizing this disconnect, perhaps the ideal method to properly delineate subclinical heart failure (HFrEF/HFpEF) should be one that takes into account ventricular function and the cardiac cycle. At present, the awareness of asymptomatic left ventricular systolic and diastolic dysfunction grows. This concept may be best represented by nomenclature such as heart failure with reduced EF with maintained cardiac output, HFrEF mCO, or with reduced cardiac output, rCO, versus heart failure with preserved EF with maintained cardiac output, HFpEF mCO, or with reduced cardiac output, rCO.

With the advent of genetics, electrocardiography, echocardiography, and cardiac imaging providers are able to phenotype patients and consider treatment options earlier in the disease course. Keeping in mind ventricular physiology, pathology, and echocardiography findings such as GLS and measuring true cardiac output may help providers hinder disease progression to clinically overt HF.

10. Conclusions

Cardiomyopathy with subclinical heart failure is a challenging and nearly impossible condition to uncover. As the awareness of this disease phenotype grows and the nuances better understood so will the early recognition of and its treatment to focus on prevention of the evolution to overt HF.

Disclosures

The authors have no relevant financial interests related to the topic of the chapter.

Author details

Hazel Contractor[1,2], Kamaldeep Singh[2,3] and Ernst von Schwarz[1,2,4,5]*

1 Cedars Sinai Medical Center, Los Angeles, California, USA

2 Dr. von Schwarz Stem Cell and Anti-Aging Institute, Beverly Hills, California, USA

3 Banner University Medical Center, University of Arizona College of Medicine, Tucson, AZ, USA

4 University of California Los Angeles (UCLA), Los Angeles, California, USA

5 Euclid University, Washington DC, USA

*Address all correspondence to: info@drvon.schwarz.com

References

[1] Brieler J, Breeden MA, Tucker J. Cardiomyopathy: An overview. American Family Physician. 2017;**96**:640-646

[2] Criteria I of M (US) C on SSCD. Heart failure, cardiomyopathy, and right heart failure. In: Cardiovascular Disability: Updating the Social Security Listings. US: National Academies Press; 2010. Available from: https://www.ncbi.nlm.nih.gov/books/NBK209980/ [Accessed: April 16, 2024]

[3] Diagnosis and Evaluation of Heart Failure | AAFP . Available from:https://www.aafp.org/pubs/afp/issues/2012/0615/p1161.html [Accessed: April 25, 2024]

[4] Kurmani S, Squire I. Acute heart failure: Definition, classification and epidemiology. Current Heart Failure Reports. 2017;**14**:385-392

[5] Ferreira A, Ferreira V, Antunes MM, Lousinha A, Pereira-da-Silva T, Antunes D, et al. Dilated cardiomyopathy: A comprehensive approach to diagnosis and risk stratification. Biomedicine. 2023;**11**:834

[6] Wang Y, Jia H, Song J. Accurate classification of non-ischemic cardiomyopathy. Current Cardiology Reports. 2023;**25**:1299-1317

[7] Charron P, Maupain C. Genetics of cardiomyopathies: Hypertrophic cardiomyopathy. In: Camm AJ, Lüscher TF, Maurer G, Serruys PW, editors. The ESC Textbook of Cardiovascular Medicine. Oxford, New York: Oxford University Press; 2018

[8] Teekakirikul P, Zhu W, Huang HC, Fung E. Hypertrophic cardiomyopathy: An overview of genetics and management. Biomolecules. 2019;**9**:878

[9] Tuohy CV, Kaul S, Song HK, Nazer B, Heitner SB. Hypertrophic cardiomyopathy: The future of treatment. European Journal of Heart Failure. 2020;**22**:228-240

[10] Palandri C, Santini L, Argirò A, Margara F, Doste R, Bueno-Orovio A, et al. Pharmacological management of hypertrophic cardiomyopathy: From bench to bedside. Drugs. 2022;**82**:889-912

[11] Mahmaljy H, Yelamanchili VS, Singhal M. Dilated Cardiomyopathy. In: StatPearls. Treasure Island (FL): StatPearls Publishing; 2024. Available from: http://www.ncbi.nlm.nih.gov/books/NBK441911/ [Accessed: April 18, 2024]

[12] Schultheiss H-P, Fairweather D, Caforio ALP, Escher F, Hershberger RE, Lipshultz SE, et al. Dilated cardiomyopathy. Nature Reviews Disease Primers. 2019;**5**:32

[13] Pinamonti B, Abate E, De Luca A, Finocchiaro G, Korcova R. Role of cardiac imaging: Echocardiography. In: Sinagra G, Merlo M, Pinamonti B, editors. Dilated Cardiomyopathy: From Genetics to Clinical Management. Cham (CH): Springer; 2019. Available from: http://www.ncbi.nlm.nih.gov/books/NBK553855/ [Accessed: April 18, 2024]

[14] Altinier A, Paldino A, Gigli M, Pappalardo A, Sinagra G. Current management and treatment. In: Sinagra G, Merlo M, Pinamonti B, editors. Dilated Cardiomyopathy: From Genetics to Clinical Management. Cham (CH): Springer; 2019. Available from: http://www.ncbi.nlm.nih.gov/books/NBK553842/ [Accessed: April 18, 2024]

[15] Brown KN, Pendela VS, Ahmed I, Diaz RR. Restrictive Cardiomyopathy.

In: StatPearls. Treasure Island (FL): StatPearls Publishing; 2024. Available from: http://www.ncbi.nlm.nih.gov/books/NBK537234/ [Accessed: April 19, 2024]

[16] Gowda SN, Ali H-J, Hussain I. Overview of restrictive cardiomyopathies. Methodist DeBakey Cardiovascular Journal. 2022;**18**:4-16

[17] Alkar BS, Mattsson G, Magnusson P, Alkar BS, Mattsson G, Magnusson P. Ischemic cardiomyopathy: Contemporary clinical management. In: Current Perspectives on Cardiomyopathies. London, UK: IntechOpen; 2018. DOI: 10.5772/intechopen.76723

[18] Bhandari B, Quintanilla Rodriguez BS, Masood W. Ischemic Cardiomyopathy. In: StatPearls. Treasure Island (FL): StatPearls Publishing; 2024. Available from: http://www.ncbi.nlm.nih.gov/books/NBK537301/ [Accessed: April 16, 2024]

[19] Muscogiuri G, Guglielmo M, Serra A, Gatti M, Volpato V, Schoepf UJ, et al. Multimodality imaging in ischemic chronic cardiomyopathy. Journal of Imaging. 2022;**8**:35

[20] Elgendy IY, Mahtta D, et al. Medical therapy for heart failure caused by ischemic heart disease. Circulation Research. 2019;**24**:1520-1535. Available from: https://www.ahajournals.org/doi/10.1161/CIRCRESAHA.118.313568#d1e408. [Accessed: April 18, 2024]

[21] Oren O, Goldberg S. Heart failure with preserved ejection fraction: Diagnosis and management. The American Journal of Medicine. 2017;**130**:510-516

[22] Pieske B et al. How to diagnose heart failure with preserved ejection fraction: The HFA–PEFF diagnostic algorithm: A consensus recommendation from the Heart Failure Association (HFA) of the European Society of Cardiology (ESC). European Journal of Heart Failure. 2020;**22**:391-412. Available from: https://academic.oup.com/eurheartj/article/40/40/3297/5557740?login=false. [Accessed: April 19, 2024]

[23] Golla MSG, Shams P. Heart failure with preserved ejection fraction (HFpEF). In: StatPearls. Treasure Island (FL): StatPearls Publishing; 2024. Available from: http://www.ncbi.nlm.nih.gov/books/NBK599960/ [Accessed: April 20, 2024]

[24] Savarese G, Stolfo D, Sinagra G, Lund LH. Heart failure with mid-range or mildly reduced ejection fraction. Nature Reviews. Cardiology. 2022;**19**:100-116

[25] Mesquita ET, Barbetta LM d S, Correia ET d O. Heart failure with mid-range ejection fraction—State of the art. Arquivos Brasileiros de Cardiologia. 2019;**112**:784-790

[26] Heidenreich P et al. 2022 AHA/ACC/HFSA guideline for the management of heart failure: A report of the American College of Cardiology/American Heart Association Joint Committee on Clinical Practice Guidelines. Circulation. 2022;**145**:e895-e1032. DOI: 10.1161/CIR.0000000000001063

[27] Schwinger RHG. Pathophysiology of heart failure. Cardiovascular Diagnosis and Therapy. 2021;**11**:263-276

[28] Hajouli S, Ludhwani D. Heart failure and ejection fraction. In: StatPearls. Treasure Island (FL): StatPearls Publishing; 2024. Available from: http://www.ncbi.nlm.nih.gov/books/NBK553115/ [Accessed: April 22, 2024]

[29] Dumitru I. Heart failure: Practice essentials, background, pathophysiology.

Heart Failure. May 2024. Published Online @TheHeart.org. Available from: https://emedicine.medscape.com/article/163062-overview?form=fpf#a3. [Accessed: April 26, 2024]

[30] Arvanitaki A, Michou E, Kalogeropoulos A, Karvounis H, Giannakoulas G. Mildly symptomatic heart failure with reduced ejection fraction: Diagnostic and therapeutic considerations. ESC Heart Failure. 2020;**7**:1477-1487

[31] Kosmala W, Marwick TH. Asymptomatic left ventricular diastolic dysfunction: Predicting progression to symptomatic heart failure. JACC: Cardiovascular Imaging. 2020;**13**:215-227

[32] Hartupee J, Mann DL. Neurohormonal activation in heart failure with reduced ejection fraction. Nature Reviews. Cardiology. 2017;**14**:30-38

[33] Sara JD, Toya T, Taher R, Lerman A, Gersh B, Anavekar NS. Asymptomatic left ventricle systolic dysfunction. European Cardiology Review. 2020;**15**:e13

[34] Echouffo-Tcheugui JB, Erqou S, Butler J, Yancy CW, Fonarow GC. Assessing the risk of progression from asymptomatic left ventricular dysfunction to overt heart failure. JACC Heart Failure. 2016;**4**:237-248

[35] McDonagh TA, Morrison CE, Lawrence A, Ford I, Tunstall-Pedoe H, McMurray JJ, et al. Symptomatic and asymptomatic left-ventricular systolic dysfunction in an urban population. The Lancet. 1997;**350**:829-833

[36] Folse R, Braunwald E. Determination of fraction of left ventricular volume ejected per beat and of ventricular end-diastolic and residual volumes: Experimental and clinical observations with a precordial dilution technic. Circulation. 1962;**25**:674-685

[37] Cingolani HE, Pérez NG, Cingolani OH, Ennis IL. The Anrep effect: 100 years later. American Journal of Physiology-Heart and Circulatory Physiology. 2013;**304**:H175-H182

[38] Patterson SW, Piper H, Starling EH. The regulation of the heart beat. The Journal of Physiology. 1914;**48**:465-513

[39] Konstam MA, Abboud FM. Ejection fraction misunderstood and overrated (changing the Paradigm in categorizing heart failure). Circulation. 2017;**135**:717-719

[40] Cikes M, Solomon SD. Beyond ejection fraction: An integrative approach for assessment of cardiac structure and function in heart failure. European Heart Journal. 2016;**37**:1642-1650

[41] Sharma S, Merghani A, Mont L. Exercise and the heart: The good, the bad, and the ugly. European Heart Journal. 2015;**36**:1445-1453

[42] Gottdiener JS, McClelland RL, Marshall R, Shemanski L, Furberg CD, Kitzman DW, et al. Outcome of congestive heart failure in elderly persons: Influence of left ventricular systolic function. Annals of Internal Medicine. 2002;**137**:631-639

[43] Curtis JP, Sokol SI, Wang Y, Rathore SS, Ko DT, Jadbabaie F, et al. The association of left ventricular ejection fraction, mortality, and cause of death in stable outpatients with heart failure. Journal of the American College of Cardiology. 2003;**42**:736-742

[44] AlJaroudi W, Alraies MC, Halley C, Rodriguez L, Grimm RA, Thomas JD, et al. Impact of progression of diastolic dysfunction on mortality in patients with Normal ejection fraction. Circulation. 2012;**125**:782-788

[45] Møller JE, Søndergaard E, Poulsen SH, Egstrup K. Pseudonormal and restrictive filling patterns predict left ventricular dilation and cardiac death after a first myocardial infarction: A serial color M-mode Doppler echocardiographic study. Journal of the American College of Cardiology. 2000;**36**:1841-1846

[46] Potter E, Marwick TH. Assessment of left ventricular function by echocardiography. JACC: Cardiovascular Imaging. 2018;**11**:260-274

[47] Kramer DG, Trikalinos TA, Kent DM, Antonpoulos GV, Konstam MA, Udelson JE. Quantitative evaluation of drug or device effects on ventricular remodeling as predictors of therapeutic effects on mortality in patients with heart failure and reduced ejection fraction: A meta-analytic approach. JACC. 2010;**56**:392-406

[48] Cikes M, Sutherland G, Anderson L, Bijnens B. The role of echocardiographic deformation imaging in hypertrophic myopathies. Nature Reviews. Cardiology. 2010;**7**:384-396

[49] Aurigemma GP, Silver KH, Priest MA, Gaasch WH. Geometric changes allow normal ejection fraction despite depressed myocardial shortening in hypertensive left ventricular hypertrophy. JACC. 1995;**26**:195-202

[50] Kraigher-Krainer E, Shah AM, Gupta DK, Santos A, Claggett B, Pieske B, et al. Impaired systolic function by strain imaging in heart failure with preserved ejection fraction. JACC. 2014;**63**:447-456

[51] Mizuguchi Y, Oishi Y, Myoshi H, Iuchi A, Nagase N, Oki T. The functional role of longitudinal, circumferential, and radial myocardial deformation for regulating the early impairment of left ventricular contraction and relaxation in patients with cardiovascular risk factors: A study with two-dimensional strain imaging. Journal of the American Society of Echocardiography. 2008;**21**:1138-1144

[52] Fang ZY, Leano R, Marwick TH. Relationship between longitudinal and radial contractility in subclinical diabetic heart disease. Clinical Science. 2004;**106**:53-60

[53] Haugaa KH, Smedsrud MK, Steen T, Kongsgaard E, Loennechen JP, Tt S, et al. Mechanical dispersion assessed by myocardial strain in patients after myocardial infarction for risk prediction of ventricular arrhythmia. JACC: Cardiovascular Imaging. 2010;**3**:247-256

[54] Wan S-H, Vogel MW, Chen HH. Pre-clinical diastolic dysfunction. Journal of the American College of Cardiology. 2014;**63**:407-416

[55] Kosmala W, Jellis CL, Marwick TH. Exercise limitation associated with asymptomatic left ventricular impairment. Journal of the American College of Cardiology. 2015;**65**:257-266

[56] Sacre JW, Wong C, Chan Y-K, Carrington MJ, Stewart S, Kingwell BA. Left ventricular dysfunction and exercise capacity trajectory. JACC: Cardiovascular Imaging. 2019;**12**:798-806

[57] Coglianese EE, Wang TJ. Clinical monitoring of stage B heart failure: Echocardiography. Heart Failure Clinics. 2012;**8**:169-178

[58] Oh JK, Borlaug BA. Stage B heart failure. Journal of the American College of Cardiology. 2015;**65**:267-269

[59] Ammar KA, Jacobsen SJ, Mahoney DW, Kors JA, Redfield MM, Burnett JC, et al. Prevalence and prognostic significance of heart failure

stages: Application of the American College of Cardiology/American Heart Association heart failure staging criteria in the community. Circulation. 2007;**115**:1563-1570

[60] Nagueh SF, Smiseth OA, Appleton CP, Byrd BF, Dokainish H, Edvardsen T, et al. Recommendations for the evaluation of left ventricular diastolic function by echocardiography: An update from the American Society of Echocardiography and the European Association of Cardiovascular Imaging. Journal of the American Society of Echocardiography. 2016;**29**:277-314

[61] Pandey A, Allen NB, Ayers C, Reis JP, Moreira HT, Sidney S, et al. Fitness in young adulthood and long-term cardiac structure and function. JACC Heart Failure. 2017;**5**:347-355

[62] Mordi IR, Singh S, Rudd A, Srinivasan J, Frenneaux M, Tzemos N, et al. Comprehensive echocardiographic and cardiac magnetic resonance evaluation differentiates among heart failure with preserved ejection fraction patients, hypertensive patients, and healthy control subjects. JACC: Cardiovascular Imaging. 2018;**11**:577-585

[63] Kosmala W, Rojek A, Przewlocka-Kosmala M, Mysiak A, Karolko B, Marwick TH. Contributions of nondiastolic factors to exercise intolerance in heart failure with preserved ejection fraction. Journal of the American College of Cardiology. 2016;**67**:659-670

[64] Yang H, Negishi K, Wang Y, Nolan M, Marwick TH. Imaging-guided Cardioprotective treatment in a community elderly population of stage B heart failure. JACC: Cardiovascular Imaging. 2017;**10**:217-226

[65] Wang Y, Yang H, Huynh Q, Nolan M, Negishi K, Marwick TH. Diagnosis of nonischemic stage B heart failure in type 2 diabetes mellitus. JACC: Cardiovascular Imaging. 2018;**11**:1390-1400

[66] Urheim S, Edvardsen T, Torp H, Angelsen B, Smiseth OA. Myocardial strain by Doppler echocardiography: Validation of a new method to quantify regional myocardial function. Circulation. 2000;**102**:1158-1164

[67] Weidemann F, Jamal F, Sutherland GR, Claus P, Kowalski M, Hatle L, et al. Myocardial function defined by strain rate and strain during alterations in inotropic states and heart rate. American Journal of Physiology-Heart and Circulatory Physiology. 2002;**283**:H792-H799

[68] Dokainish H, Sengupta R, Pillai M, Bobek J, Lakkis N. Assessment of left ventricular systolic function using echocardiography in patients with preserved ejection fraction and elevated diastolic pressures. The American Journal of Cardiology. 2008;**101**:1766-1771

[69] Tan YT, Wenzelburger F, Lee E, Heatlie G, Patel K, Frenneaux M, et al. The pathophysiology of heart failure with normal ejection fraction: Exercise echocardiography reveals complex abnormalities of both systolic and diastolic ventricular function involving torsion, untwist, and longitudinal motion. JACC. 2009;**54**:36-46

[70] Aurigemma GP, Zile MR, Gaasch WH. Contractile behavior of the left ventricle in diastolic heart failure: With emphasis on regional systolic function. Circulation. 2006;**113**:296-304

[71] Vinereanu D, Lim PO, Frenneaux MP, Fraser AG. Reduced myocardial velocities of left ventricular long-axis contraction identify both systolic and diastolic heart failure-a comparison with brain natriuretic peptide. European Heart Journal. 2005;**7**:512-519

[72] Bruch C, Gradus R, Gunia S, Breithardt G, Wichter T. Doppler tissue analysis of mitral annular velocities: Evidence for systolic abnormalities in patients with diastolic heart failure. Journal of the American Society of Echocardiography. 2003;**16**:1031-1036

[73] Yip GW, Zhang Q, Xie J-M, Liang Y-J, Liu Y-M, Yan B, et al. Resting global and regional left ventricular contractility in patients with heart failure and normal ejection fraction: Insights from speckle-tracking echocardiography. Heart. 2011;**97**:287-294

[74] Wang J, Khoury DS, Yue Y, Torre-Amione G, Nagueh SF. Preserved left ventricular twist and circumferential deformation, but depressed longitudinal and radial deformation in patients with diastolic heart failure. European Heart Journal. 2007;**29**:1283-1289

[75] Shah AM, Solomon SD. Phenotypic and pathophysiological heterogeneity in heart failure with preserved ejection fraction. European Heart Journal. 2012;**33**:171-1717

[76] Shah AM, Claggett B, Sweitzer N, Shah SJ, Anand IS, Liu L, et al. Prognostic importance of impaired systolic function in heart failure with preserved ejection fraction and the impact of spironolactone clinical perspective. Circulation. 2015;**132**:402-414

[77] Libby P, Bonow RO, Mann DL, Tomaselli GF, Bhatt D, Solomon SD, et al. Braunwald's Heart Disease: A Textbook of Cardiovascular Medicine. 12th ed. Amsterdam, Oxford, London, New York: Elsevier; 2021. pp. 1-1902

[78] Zipes DP, Camm AJ, Borggrefe M, Buxton AE, Chaitman B, Fromer M, et al. Guidelines for management of patients with ventricular arrhythmias and the prevention of sudden cardiac death: A report of the American College of Cardiology/American Heart Association task force and the European Society of Cardiology Committee for practice guidelines (writing committee to develop guidelines for Management of Patients with Ventricular Arrhythmias and the prevention of sudden cardiac death): *Developed in collaboration with the European heart rhythm association and the Heart Rhythm Society*. Circulation. 2006;**2006**:114. DOI: 10.1161/CIRCULATIONAHA.106.178233

[79] Goldberger JJ, Cain ME, Hohnloser SH, Kadish AH, Knight BP, Lauer MS, et al. American Heart Association/American College of Cardiology Foundation/Heart Rhythm Society scientific statement on noninvasive risk stratification techniques for identifying patients at risk for sudden cardiac death: A scientific statement from the American Heart Association Council on clinical cardiology committee on electrocardiography and arrhythmias and council on epidemiology and prevention. Circulation. 2008;**118**:1497-1518

[80] Kristensen SL, Castagno D, Shen L, Jhund P, Docherty K, Rorth R, et al. Prevalence and incidence of intraventricular conduction delays and outcomes in patients with heart failure and reduced ejection fraction: Insights from PARADIGM-HF and ATMOSPHERE. European Journal of Heart Failure. 2020;**22**:2370-2379

[81] Kirk JA, Kass DA. Cellular and molecular aspects of dyssynchrony and resynchronization. Cardiac Electrophysiology Clinical. 2015;7:585-597

[82] Hussein AA, Wilkoff BL. Cardiac implantable electronic device therapy in heart failure. Circulation Research. 2019;**124**:1584-1597

[83] Abraham WT, Adamson PB, Bourge RC, Aaron MF, Costanzo MR,

Stevenson LW, et al. Wireless pulmonary artery haemodynamic monitoring in chronic heart failure: A randomised controlled trial. The Lancet. 2011;**377**:658-666

[84] Hasenfub G, Hayward C, Burkhoff D, Silvestry FE, McKenzie S, Gusafsson F, et al. A transcatheter intracardiac shunt device for heart failure with preserved ejection fraction (REDUCE LAP-HF): A multicentre, open-label, single-arm, phase 1 trial. The Lancet. 2016;**387**:1298-1304

[85] Feldman T, Mauri L, Kahwash R, Litwin S, Ricciardi MJ, Van Der Harst P, et al. Transcatheter interatrial shunt device for the treatment of heart failure with preserved ejection fraction (REDUCE LAP-HF I [Reduce elevated left atrial pressure in patients with heart failure]): A phase 2, randomized, sham-controlled trial. Circulation. 2018;**137**:364-375

[86] Tschope C, Kherad B, Klein O, Lipp A, Blaschke F, Gutterman D, et al. Cardiac contractility modulation: Mechanisms of action in heart failure with reduced ejection fraction and beyond. European Journal of Heart Failure. 2018;**21**:14-22

[87] Borggrefe M, Burkhoff D. Clinical effects of cardiac contractility modulation (CCM) as a treatment for chronic heart failure. European Journal of Heart Failure. 2012;**14**:703-712

[88] Kuschyk J, Kloppe A, Schmidt-Schweda S, Bonnemeier H, Röger S. Cardiac contractility modulation: A technical guide for device implantation. Reviews in Cardiovascular Medicine. 2017;**18**:1-13

[89] Rastogi S, Mishra S, Zacà V, Mika Y, Rousso B, Sabbah HN. Effects of chronic therapy with cardiac contractility modulation electrical signals on cytoskeletal proteins and matrix metalloproteinases in dogs with heart failure. Cardiology. 2008;**110**:230-237

[90] Zhang Q, Chan Y-S, Liang Y-J, Fang F, Lam Y-Y, Chan C-P, et al. Comparison of left ventricular reverse remodeling induced by cardiac contractility modulation and cardiac resynchronization therapy in heart failure patients with different QRS durations. International Journal of Cardiology. 2013;**167**:889-893

[91] Butter C, Wellnhofer E, Schlegl M, Winbeck G, Fleck E, Sabbah HN. Enhanced inotropic state of the failing left ventricle by cardiac contractility modulation electrical signals is not associated with increased myocardial oxygen consumption. Journal of Cardiac Failure. 2007;**13**:137-142

[92] Patel PA, Nadarajah R, Ali N, Gierula J, Witte KK. Cardiac contractility modulation for the treatment of heart failure with reduced ejection fraction. Heart Failure Reviews. 2021;**26**:217-226

[93] Yu C-M, Chan JY-S, Zhang Q, Yip GWK, Lam Y-Y, Chan A, et al. Impact of cardiac contractility modulation on left ventricular global and regional function and remodeling. JACC: Cardiovascular Imaging. 2009;**2**:1341-1349

[94] Vartanian K, Franco M, Busse N, Bidzhoian S, Hamdan T, von Schwarz ER. Improved physical function after cardiac contractility modulation therapy in 10 patients with chronic heart failure. Texas Heart Institute Journal. 2022;**49**:e227905

[95] Costanzo MR, Ponikowski P, Javaheri S, Augostini R, Goldberg L, Holcomb R, et al. Transvenous neurostimulation for central sleep apnoea: A randomised controlled trial. The Lancet. 2016;**388**:974-982

[96] Eulenburg C, Wegscheider K, Woehrle H, Angermann C, d'Ortho M-P, Erdmann E, et al. Mechanisms underlying increased mortality risk in patients with heart failure and reduced ejection fraction randomly assigned to adaptive servoventilation in the SERVE-HF study: Results of a secondary multistate modelling analysis. The Lancet Respiratory Medicine. 2016;**4**:873-881

[97] Sobowale C, Hori Y, Ajijola O. Neuromodulation therapy in heart failure: Combined use of drugs and devices. Journal of Innovations Cardiac Rhythm Management. 2020;**11**:4151-4159

[98] Zile MR, Abraham WT, Weaver FA, Butter C, Ducharme A, Halbach M, et al. Baroreflex activation therapy for the treatment of heart failure with a reduced ejection fraction: Safety and efficacy in patients with and without cardiac resynchronization therapy. European Journal of Heart Failure. 2015;**17**:1066-1074

[99] Zile MR, Abraham WT, Lindenfeld J, Weaver FA, Zannad F, Graves T, et al. First granted example of novel FDA trial design under expedited access pathway for premarket approval: BeAT-HF. American Heart Journal. 2018;**204**:139-150

[100] Shore S, Grau-Sepulveda MV, Bhatt DL, Heidenreich PA, Eapen ZJ, Hernandez AF, et al. Characteristics, treatments, and outcomes of hospitalized heart failure patients stratified by etiologies of cardiomyopathy. JACC Heart Failure. 2015;**3**:906-916

[101] Velazquez EJ, Lee KL, Jones RH, Al-Khalidi HR, Hill JA, Panza JA, et al. Coronary-artery bypass surgery in patients with ischemic cardiomyopathy. The New England Journal of Medicine. 2016;**374**:1511-1520

[102] Rush C, Berry C, Oldroyd K, Rocchiccioli P, Lindsay M, Campbell R, et al. Prevalence of coronary artery disease and coronary microvascular dysfunction in heart failure with preserved ejection fraction. European Heart Journal. 2019;**40**:ehz747.0043

[103] Mohammed SF, Hussain S, Mirzoyev SA, Edwards WD, Maleszewski JJ, Redfield MM. Coronary microvascular rarefaction and myocardial fibrosis in heart failure with preserved ejection fraction. Circulation. 2015;**131**:550-559

[104] Hwang S-J, Melenovsky V, Borlaug BA. Implications of coronary artery disease in heart failure with preserved ejection fraction. Journal of the American College of Cardiology. 2014;**63**:2817-2827

[105] Chehab O, Roberts-Thomson R, Ng Yin Ling C, Marber M, Prendergast BD, Rajani R, et al. Secondary mitral regurgitation: Pathophysiology, proportionality and prognosis. Heart. 2020;**106**:716-723

[106] Park K-H, Jeong MH, Lee MG, Ko JS, Sim DS, Yoon NS, et al. What is the optimal duration of triple anti-platelet therapy in patients with acute myocardial infarction undergoing drug-eluting stent implantation? Journal of Cardiology. 2011;**57**:53-60

[107] Kaneko H, Kiriyama H, Kamon T, Itoh H, Kodera S, Fujiu K, et al. Percutaneous mitral valve intervention using MitraClip for functional mitral regurgitation and heart failure. International Heart Journal. 2021;**62**:4-8

[108] Vahanian A, Beyersdorf F, Praz F, Milojevic M, Baldus S, Bauersachs J, et al. 2021 ESC/EACTS guidelines for the management of valvular heart disease: Developed by the task force for the

management of valvular heart disease of the European Society of Cardiology (ESC) and the European Association for Cardio-Thoracic Surgery (EACTS). Revista Espanola Cardiologia Engl Ed. 2022;**75**:524

[109] Feldman T, Kar S, Elmariah S, Smart SC, Trento A, Siegel RJ, et al. Randomized comparison of percutaneous repair and surgery for mitral regurgitation. Journal of the American College of Cardiology. 2015;**66**:2844-2854

[110] Stone GW, Lindenfeld J, Abraham WT, Kar S, Lim DS, Mishell JM, et al. Transcatheter mitral-valve repair in patients with heart failure. The New England Journal of Medicine. 2018;**379**:2307-2318

[111] Yancy CW, Jessup M, Bozkurt B, Butler J, Casey DE, Drazner MH, et al. ACCF/AHA guideline for the management of heart failure: A report of the American College of Cardiology Foundation/American Heart Association task Force on Practice Guidelines. Circulation. 2013;**2013**:128. DOI: 10.1161/CIR.0b013e31829e8776

[112] Russo MJ. Pretransplantation patient characteristics and survival following combined heart and kidney transplantation: An analysis of the united network for organ sharing database. Archives of Surgery. 2009;**144**:241

[113] Shah MR, Starling RC, Schwartz Longacre L, Mehra MR. Heart transplantation research in the next decade—A goal to achieving evidence-based outcomes. Journal of the American College of Cardiology. 2012;**59**:1263-1269

[114] Mehra M, Kobashigawa J, Starling R, Russell S, Uber P, Parameshwar J, et al. Listing criteria for heart transplantation: International Society for Heart and Lung Transplantation Guidelines for the Care of Cardiac Transplant Candidates—2006. The Journal of Heart and Lung Transplantation. 2006;**25**:1024-1042

[115] Stehlik J, Edwards LB, Kucheryavaya AY, Benden C, Christie JD, Dobbels F, et al. The registry of the International Society for Heart and Lung Transplantation: Twenty-eighth adult heart transplant report—2011. The Journal of Heart and Lung Transplantation. 2011;**30**:1078-1094

[116] Starling RC. Advanced heart failure: Transplantation, LVADs, and beyond. Cleveland Clinic Journal of Medicine. 2013;**80**:33-40

[117] Taylor DO, Stehlik J, Edwards LB, Aurora P, Christie JD, Dobbels F, et al. Registry of the International Society for Heart and Lung Transplantation: Twenty-sixth official adult heart transplant report—2009. The Journal of Heart and Lung Transplantation. 2009;**28**:1007-1022

[118] Phan TT, Shivu GN, Abozguia K, Davies C, Nassimizadeh M, Jimenez D, et al. Impaired heart rate recovery and chronotropic incompetence in patients with heart failure with preserved ejection fraction. Circulation. Heart Failure. 2010;**3**:29-34

[119] Shah SJ. Precision medicine for heart failure with preserved ejection fraction: An overview. Journal of Cardiovascular Translational Research. 2017;**10**:233-244

Chapter 5

Diabetes-Induced Cardiomyopathy: Updates in Epidemiology, Prevention, and Management

Ernest A. Adeghate, Sahar Mohsin, Ahmed Bin Amar, Suhail AlAmry, Mariam AlOtaiba, Omobola Awosika Oyeleye and Jaipaul Singh

Abstract

Diabetes mellitus (DM) is a condition of abnormal carbohydrate metabolism, leading to persistent hyperglycemia. It is defined as a fasting blood glucose over 7.0 mmol/L, a 2-hour plasma post-meal of 11.1 mmol/L, or HbA1C values over 6.5% (48 mmol/L). DM affects almost 600 million people globally with an annual cost of around three trillion US dollars. These data indicate that DM is a global health burden that warrants attention. Complications of DM include nephropathy, retinopathy, neuropathy, and cardiomyopathy. DM-induced hyperglycemia causes oxidative stress, inflammation, endothelial and mitochondrial abnormality, and subsequently, cardiomyopathy. Hyperglycemia stimulates many signaling pathways including polyol, and hexokinase, resulting in the formation of vascular endothelial lesions, free radicals and carbonyl anions, transforming growth factor-β1, fibronectin, and nuclear factor kappa-B, which increase fibrosis and inflammation in the myocardium. All of these pathological processes lead to defective vascular permeability and hypoxia in cardiac tissue, ischemia, and eventually heart failure, and sudden cardiac death. The onset of diabetic cardiomyopathy could be delayed with a healthy lifestyle (balanced diet, physical activity, sleep, low stress, non-smoking). GLP-1 receptor agonists with or without SGLT2i are beneficial additions for the treatment of diabetic cardiomyopathy.

Keywords: diabetes mellitus, complications of diabetes, cardiomyopathy, heart failure, prevention, management, anti-diabetic drugs, myocardial remodeling, gender, ethnicity, disability and quality of life

1. Introduction

1.1 Diabetes (DM): epidemiology and associated complications

DM is a complex condition currently having an impact on over 600 million individuals aged 20–78 years worldwide, with 250 million undiagnosed and 2 billion with prediabetes [1, 2]. The disorder is divided into two main groups: Type 1 diabetes mellitus (T1-DM) and Type 2 or non-insulin dependent diabetes (T2-DM). T1-DM arises by the demolition of the endocrine β-cells of the islet of Langerhans by immune cells, resulting in inadequate insulin release, while T2-DM is due to lifestyle habits including unhealthy diets and physical inactivity. This results in insulin resistance (IR) where insulin molecules cannot be imbibed into skeletal muscle. DM is now a global pandemic with a global widespread presence that will rise to 800 million people in 2045 [1, 3].

The annual cost of treating and managing diabetic patients in 2021 in the US was estimated at one trillion US dollars and three trillion US dollars globally [4]. The high prevalence and the amount of funds for managing DM and its associated complications have posed severe distress to healthcare providers and individuals with the disorder worldwide (**Table 1**).

The ten nations with the highest widespread occurrence of diabetes mellitus, from the highest to lowest, are: Pakistan-Islamic Republic (30.80%), Kuwait-State (24.90%), Republic of Nauru (23.40%), New Caledonia Islands (23.40%), Islands of Northern Mariana (23.40%), Marshall Islands of the US (23.00%), Republic of Mauritius (22.60%), Arab Republic of Egypt (20.90%), Qatar (19.50%), Malaysia (19.00%) [1]. Unfortunately, most of the increases in the number of people with DM are found in poorer countries.

		DM cases in 2021 (millions)	**Projected DM cases in 2045 (millions)**	**% Increase from 2021 to 2045**	**Ref**
1	Worldwide	537	784	46	[1]
2	Africa (Nigeria, South Africa, Kenya, etc.)	24	55	134	[1]
3	South-East Asia (India, Bangladesh, Indonesia, etc.)	90	152	68	[1]
4	Europe (UK, France, Germany, Italy, etc.)	61	69	13	[1]
5	North America & Caribbean (United States of America, Mexico, Canada, etc.)	51	63	24	[1]
6	Middle East & North Africa (Egypt, Pakistan, Iran, Saudi Arabia, Sudan, etc.)	73	136	87	[5]
7	South and Central America (Brazil, Argentina, Chile, etc.)	32	49	50	
8	Western Pacific (China, Japan, Australia, Philippines, Malaysia, Vietnam, etc.)	206	260	27	

WHO = World Health Organization.

Table 1.
The pattern of distribution of diabetes mellitus type 2 cases among those between the ages of 20 and 79 years, in different WHO zones in 2021 and 2045 (projected).

1.2 Gender, ethnicity, and diabetic cardiomyopathy

Diabetes affects ethnic groups differentially, striking some ethnic groups more severely than others. For example, the Pima Indians of the USA acquire T2-DM at a rate that is double that seen in Caucasians. Other ethnic groups that are also at higher risk include Latinos, Asians, and African Americans [5].

Several epidemiological investigations have indicated that the widespread occurrence of T2-DM is four times in people from South Asian countries compared to Caucasians. In addition, people from Southern Asia nations become diabetic at an earlier age compared to Caucasians [6]. Women with DM, on the other hand, are relatively more susceptible to developing cardiovascular events when compared to men [7]. The reason for this is unknown, but hormonal interference may contribute to this difference. Since DM is as twice as high in Pima Indians compared to Caucasians, the prevalence of DCM will most likely be higher in this ethnic group.

The reasons for these ethnic differences may be due to some or all of the following: a): access to optimal health care, b): standard of living, c): awareness about illnesses in general and DM in particular, d): social coherence, e): eating habits, and f): physical exercise. In addition to genetics and environmental factors, it is also likely that the opportunity to use health services and other social factors that determine health (SDOH) could explain some of the disparities in the pathophysiological manifestations and severity of DM and its associated complications [8].

The majority of Caucasians will likely have better access to the above-listed items compared to their non-Caucasian counterparts.

Other ethnic groups including Latinos, Asians, and African Americans are more likely to develop DM and its complications (including DCM) when compared to their Caucasian counterparts [8]. It is worth noting, however, that inherited and modifiable external factors also contribute to the pathogenicity and severity of DM, and its associated co-morbidities and complications [8].

2. Pathophysiological considerations in diabetic cardiomyopathy

DM is a dysfunction of the pancreas to regulate the metabolism of carbohydrates. The inability of insulin to effectively control carbohydrate metabolism also leads to disturbances in lipid, and protein metabolisms, also associated with diabetic cardiomyopathy [3, 8]. **Figure 1** illustrates the pathological pathways leading to diabetic cardiomyopathy (DCM). 35–50% of all cases of cardiomyopathies cause arrhythmias, HF, and subsequently, SCD (sudden death of the heart).

Many factors put people at risk of getting T2DM. They include unhealthy diets, obesity or overweight, aging, genetic factors, physical inactivity, ethnicity, polycystic ovary syndrome, and others. These risk factors can act synergistically to elicit diabetes-induced hyperglycemia (HG). HG is the insulting factor, which works in tandem with protein and lipid metabolic pathways to generate certain reactive species that induce oxidative stress (OS). OS has a direct insulting, and damaging effect on mitochondria, cells, nerves, and tissues within the myocardium. These eventually precipitate a reduced heart rate and force of contraction.

These pathological processes are due to derangements in cation-transporting proteins, and contractile proteins, thereby compromising the excitation-contraction (ECC) process. With time, the myocardium develops diastolic dysfunction due to

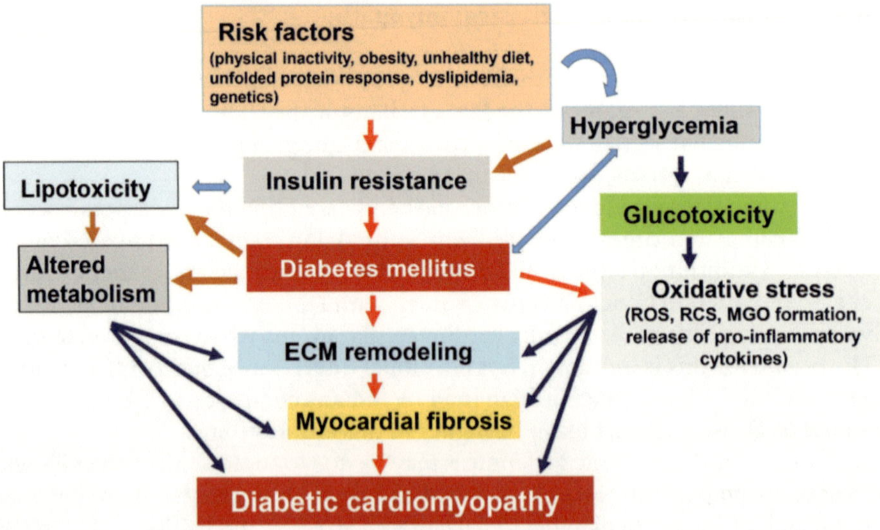

Figure 1.
Illustrates the pathological conditions contributing to the initiation of diabetic cardiomyopathy. ROS = Reactive oxygen free radical species; RCS = reactive carbonyl free radical species; MGO = methylglyoxal.

delayed contraction and relaxation (filling), reduced cardiac output, and subsequently arrhythmias, HF, and SCD [9–12].

This review will now concentrate on how hyperglycemia can induce structural changes in the myocardium, OS (oxidative stress) and inflammation, lesions of the mitochondria and endothelial lining, cardiac energy metabolism, extracellular matrix (ECM), and development of cardiac fibrosis, remodeling of the heart and abnormalities in calcium signaling and contractile proteins. In addition, the review will describe the roles of potential biochemical markers, signature proteins, and other factors associated with the development of DCM, since they play significant roles in its development. **Figure 1** shows the different pathological events leading to diabetic cardiomyopathy. These events include, but are not limited to, hyperglycemia, insulin resistance emanating from obesity, unfolded protein response, physical inactivity, and dyslipidemia. Hyperglycemia can cause glucotoxicity and OS that enhance extracellular matrix restructuring, myocardium fibrosis, and eventually DCM.

3. DM-induced oxidative stress, inflammatory chain reaction, and dysfunction of mitochondria

T2-DM-induced hyperglycemia (HG) leads to oxidative stress and inflammatory reactions, which elicit a switch of metabolic homeostatic processes in the heart leading to glucose intolerance. Mitochondrial damage leads to the overproduction of ROS and RCS in diabetic subjects leading to increased fatty oxidation and lipotoxicity in cardiomyocytes. This is coupled with increased levels of superoxide anion radicals, AGE (advanced-glycation-end-products), and enhancement of the receptors for AGE.

These oxidants also induce oxidative distress within the mitochondrion culminating in disaggregation, reduction in number, height, length, and width, and

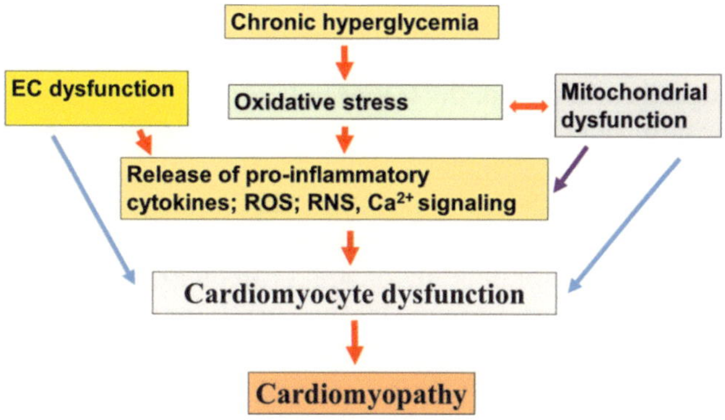

Figure 2.
Pathophysiology of hyperglycemic-induced cardiac damage. EC = Cells of the endothelium cell; ROS = Reactive oxygen free radical species; RNS = Reactive nitrogen free radical species.

formation of blebs or vesicles and marked elevation in cristae number to compensate for mitochondria damage, and loss in DCM [13–16]. It is now well established that mitochondria damage and dysfunction are determinant factors in the development of cardiac insufficiency-progression, and subsequently, diabetes-induced cardiomyopathy. This pathophysiological event is due to abnormally elevated high-energy phosphates release and increased production of ROS and RCS [17]. Once the mitochondrion is in distress due to damage by oxidants such as ROS and RNS and unable to produce energy, the myocyte and conductive tissue damage ensues [12, 14, 18].

3.1 How do chronic hyperglycemia and oxidative stress induce cardiomyocyte dysfunction?

It is paramount to stress the effect of chronic HG, a major sign of DM, in the initiation of cardiomyocyte dysfunction. HG induces oxidative stress (OS) at the cellular, tissue, and systemic levels. The OS induced by HG can then cause the release of several noxious biological factors such as cytokines that promote inflammation, ROS, and RCS [19, 20]. In addition, calcium and other signaling pathways are impaired after the onset of DM. These factors, in addition to other DM-induced pathologies, contribute to the dysfunction of the cardiomyocyte that eventually leads to the development of DCM (**Figure 2**).

4. Endothelial cell dysfunction in DM

The endothelium maintains homeostasis of the vascular bed through blood flow regulation, and vascular tone, and prevents bleeding and thrombosis formation [21]. The endothelial cells (ECs) are located on the endothelial layer or the internal tunic of blood vessels. Therefore, any pathological changes in the EC may result in abnormal function in ECs, leading to vascular disease of the myocardium [22, 23]. When the endothelium within the myocardium is exposed to chronic hyperglycemia due to diabetes, it induces a cascade of dysfunctions leading to the induction of myocardial diseases including diabetes-induced cardiomyopathy [23, 24].

5. Derangement in calcium signaling in DM

Diabetes-induced cardiomyopathy (DCM) is a major pathological disease of the heart, where cardiomyocytes become weak and frail. DCM also damages the conductive tissues and cation-transporting proteins in the heart [12, 25]. Hyperglycemia generates oxidants such as ROS and RCS, which have direct adverse effects on the homeostasis of cellular calcium and other cations including potassium. Calcium is the second messenger, initiator, modulator, and promoter of the coupling excitation-contraction process in the myocardium [11, 14, 22, 23]. It has been shown that the coupling process can be damaged by factors such as hyperglycemia associated with DM [11, 14, 25–28].

Methylglyoxal (MGO), an α-di-carbonyl RCS, is the main inducer of "carbonyl stress" [14, 29]. RCS are free radicals (reactive molecules) that cause conformational changes to biological macromolecules through AGE action [14, 30]. RCS, ROS, and RNS impair cell organelle function to induce autophagy and apoptosis [29–32].

The dysfunction of RyR and SERCA to regulate cytosolic calcium transport during diabetes leads to an elevation in diastolic calcium, which in turn results in delayed contraction and relaxation of the heart. These events play a part in the initiation of heart diseases like cardiomyopathy [14, 33]. Recent studies have revealed that gene therapy can be used successfully to delay the occurrence of diabetes-induced cardiomyopathy by targeting the synthesis of the glyoxylate-1 enzyme that breaks down MGO, a major RCS in the myocardium [33]. There is also evidence that regular daily exercise can control diabetes by increasing the beta cell mass of the endocrine pancreas and insulin release [34]. In addition to gene therapy and daily exercise, it is equally important to develop novel drugs to inhibit vascular adhesion protein that synthesizes MGO and other drugs, which can inhibit the breakdown of glyoxylase-1.

6. Extracellular matrix (ECM) development (fibrosis) and remodeling of the myocardium in DM

Most of the morbid and mortal events associated with DM are due to the DM-induced conditions of the cardiovascular apparatus such as the disease of the blood vessels supplying the heart and DCM [35]. Fibrosis, observed in the diabetic heart, is a biochemically induced morphological process, which involves the excessive tissue levels of ECM components. These components include fibrin, fibrinogen, fibronectin, laminins, collagens, elastin, myosin, and other connective tissue matrices. The accumulation of these ECM components can contribute to organ dysfunctions [10, 36].

HG, lipotoxicity, and insulin resistance (IR) activate molecules responsible for the deposition of fibers in the myocardium.

DM-induced hyperglycemia can also stimulate several fibrogenic pathways to generate ROS and RCS to induce neurohumoral responses and activate growth factor formation and downstream cascades. One such major growth factor is TGF-β1, which can induce the enlargement of the myocardium and upregulate fibro-genic matricellular proteins to form more pronounced and clinically significant fibrosis [13, 35, 36].

DOI: http://dx.doi.org/10.5772/intechopen.1006679

Diabetes-induced fibrosis impairs the contractile function and the electrophysiological properties of the heart, resulting in ventricular stiffness, delayed conduction, heart failure/cardiomyopathy, arrhythmogenesis, and SCD [36].

At an earlier stage of all these events, the myocardium undergoes a physiological remodeling process to enable the pumping of blood until the organ is repaired naturally or treated with drugs.

7. Other metabolic factors and protein signatures associated with diabetes-induced cardiomyopathy

Several metabolic factors, signature proteins, biomarkers, and cellular mediators contribute to the pathogenesis of DCM. This section briefly describes the involvement of these components. **Figure 3** illustrates the roles of some typical metabolic factors, signature proteins, biomarkers, and cellular mediators in the progression of DCM. The renin angiotensin aldosterone system abbreviated as RAAS is enhanced in people with DM [37]. The RAAS in turn stimulates NF-κB release. This promotes the release of TNF-alpha, MCP-1, IL-6, and IL-8 [38, 39]. DM promotes increased tissue levels of NF-κB in the myocardium to increase NADP oxidase-mediated release of ROS, superoxide, and peroxynitrite radicals. This process consumes the available nitric oxide, an important signaling molecular for the vasculature of the myocardium. Abnormal profiles of cAMP-responsive element modulator [40], free fatty acid [41], transcription factor Nrf2 [42], PKC (protein kinase-C) [19], cardiac Poly(ADP-ribose) polymerase 1 [43], miRNA [44], MAPK and JNK [45], SGLT2 [46], AMPK [46], O-GlcNAC [46], and autonomic neuropathy [47] also take part in determining whether DCM occurs (**Figure 3**).

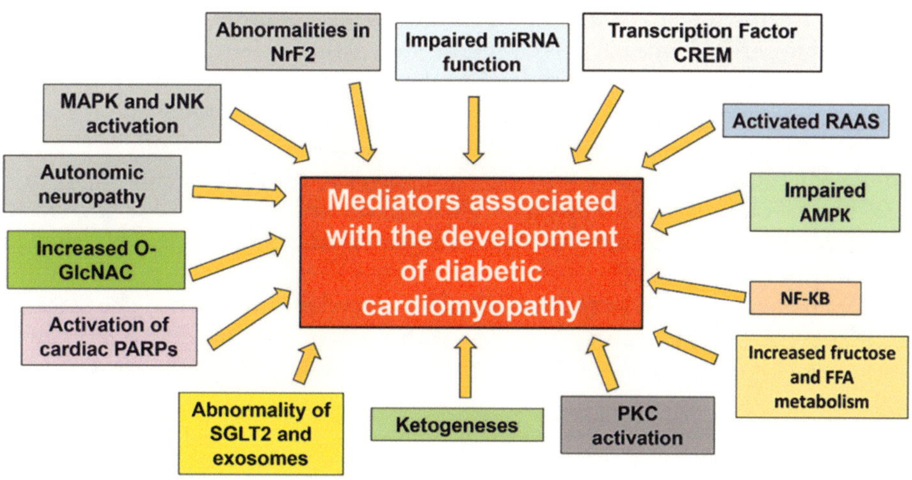

Figure 3.
Signature proteins and other biomarkers implicated in the etiopathogenesis of DCM. CREM = cAMP-responsive element modulator, FFA = Free fatty acid, NrF2 = nuclear factor erythroid 2-related-factor-2; PKC = protein kinase-C.

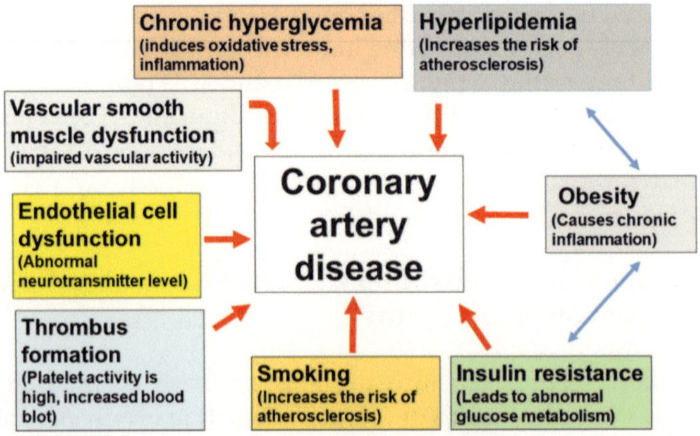

Figure 4.
Factors leading to the initiation of diabetes-induced coronary artery lesions.

8. How does diabetes mellitus contribute to coronary artery disease?

T2-DM predisposes patients to developing coronary artery disease (CAD). Indeed, it is estimated that people with T2-DM are more likely to have CAD [48, 49]. As described earlier, people with DM have an increased tendency for atherosclerosis. There are many factors, which predispose diabetic patients to developing atherosclerosis. These factors include insulin resistance, chronic hyperglycemia, elevated plasma concentrations of lipid molecules, OS, inflammatory reactions, and the dysfunction of EC, the coagulation process, and vascular smooth muscle [50–52]. Many other elements of dysmetabolic syndrome, like obesity, and high blood pressure also contribute to the etiology of CAD [53–55].

Severe obesity, IR, and chronic hyperglycemia enhance the release of inflammatory cytokines. Obesity, by itself, can induce many of the components (DM, hyperlipidemia, atherosclerosis, cardiovascular diseases) of Syndrome-X [56, 57]. These factors and hyperlipidemia hasten the deposition of atherosclerotic plaques in blood vessels [58] including coronary arteries. The deposition of lipid- and macrophage-laden plaques causes stenosis of the blood vessels of the heart bringing about a poor blood flow to the myocardial layer of the heart. Insufficient blood supply to the myocardium will cause hypoxia and injury of cardiomyocytes. All of these are risk factors for DCM. DM causes impaired blood coagulation, leading to increased formation of micro-thrombi in coronary arteries because of the enhanced function of platelets and the affinity of blood to clot [59].

In DM patients, there is an elevated circulating level of osteonectin. The plasma level of osteonectin has a direct correlation with the manifestation and severity of atherosclerotic deposition in coronary artery endothelium [60, 61] **Figure 4**.

9. Prevention of diabetes (DM) and diabetic cardiomyopathy (DCM)

The surest way to avoid DCM is to prevent DM. There are numerous ways and activities that, if applied effectively, can delay the onset of DM and hence DCM **Table 2**.

		Effect on DM/DCM	Ref
1	Healthy and balanced diet	Reduces blood glucose and HbA1c levels.	[62, 63]
2	Physical activity: aerobic and anaerobic	Increases insulin sensitivity and reduces blood glucose and HbA1c levels.	[3]
3	Sleep	Loss of sleep increases blood glucose level.	[64]
4	Reduction of stress	Stress increases blood glucose level.	[65]
5	Avoid cigarette smoking	Increases blood glucose via nicotine.	[66]
6	Avoid excessive alcohol intake	Increases in blood glucose levels in well-nourished individuals may cause pancreatitis.	[67]
7	Weight reduction	Improves diabetes signs and cardiac functions.	[68–69]
8	Hypoglycemic agents	Reduces blood glucose level.	[70–74]

Table 2.
List of activities that can help to prevent and/or manage diabetic cardiomyopathy.

9.1 Healthy and balanced diet

A healthy and well-balanced diet will deliver the necessary micronutrients, vitamins, proteins, and carbohydrates required for normal body function. A diet with a lot of greens, nuts, and fresh fruits, with a balanced proportion of protein, carbohydrates, and fat, will not only bring the needed micronutrients and trace elements but an optimal dose of energy to complete our daily tasks. Micronutrients and trace elements, including zinc and magnesium, are crucial for the function of several enzymes and biological pathways that regulate our energy homeostasis. The fine regulation of energy homeostasis determines whether an individual becomes diabetic. Literature reports have indicated that a balanced and individualized diet may reduce the level of HbA1c in diabetic patients [62, 63].

9.2 Physical activity

Physical activity such as resistance, aerobic exercise, and high-intensity interval exercise can reduce the body's total weight and increase the body's sensitivity to insulin and blood glucose in DM patients. The prospect of developing DCM is grossly reduced if the blood sugar concentration is optimal. In addition, long-term physical exercise (PE) can increase the mass of skeletal musculature. Since voluntary muscle cells uptake glucose molecules, increased skeletal muscle mass and activity will consume blood glucose levels, thereby lowering plasma sugar concentration [3]. PE also increases fat oxidation and reduces fat deposition in both the hepatic and adipose tissues. PE also reduces triglycerides and inflammation in tissues, both of which can complicate the management of DM and CDM [3].

9.3 Sleep

Adequate sleep has long been shown to contribute to optimal glucose homeostasis. During the sleep phase, blood glucose levels remain fairly constant. However, loss of sleep leads to abnormal glucose metabolism, more appetite for food, and a tendency to eat any type of food, and more time available to consume food [64]. All of these indicate that loss of sleep could result in poor sugar control and worsen the outcome of DM and DCM. Therefore, a crucial part of the management of DM must not be limited to the ingestion of food or pharmaceutical treatment alone, it must include lifestyle patterns such as sleep deprivation and sleep cycles.

9.4 Reduction of stress

Several reports have shown that diabetes can be induced by either psychological or physical stress. Stress, through the activation of the nervous systems, can increase the level of stress hormones including but not limited to catecholamines and glucocorticoids. These hormones are known inducers of insulin resistance [65]. These hormones can also increase blood glucose level leading to chronic hyperglycemia, with a sequelae of oxidative stress. All of these factors lead to a more severe DCM. Therefore, clinicians and advocates must investigate the relationship between the onset and complications of DM and the stressors in the lives of their patients or clients.

9.5 Cigarette smoking

In one experiment examining the effect of cigarette smoking on diabetes, a group of 26 diabetic and 24 non-diabetic subjects were asked to smoke two sticks of cigarettes. The plasma sugar concentrations were later measured before cigarette smoking and at 15, 30, and 60 min post cigarette smoking. These observations suggest that the blood sugar level increased markedly after cigarette smoking in both control, non-diabetic, and diabetic groups, but more profound in diabetic subjects. The culprit for the increase in blood glucose levels is nicotine, which has been reported to stimulate the release of hormones (catecholamines, glucocorticoids) capable of increasing the circulating blood level of glucose [66]. In addition to all other known cardiac-related consequences of cigarette smoking, patients with diabetes must be informed about their heightened risk of complications.

9.6 Excessive alcohol intake

Excessive intake of alcohol increases blood glucose levels in well-fed diabetic patients. In contrast, it may cause hypoglycemia in a poorly nourished diabetic patient. In addition, excessive alcohol consumption can lead to the occurrence of hypertriglyceridemia and vascular (retinopathy, neuropathy) diseases of diabetes [67]. Therefore, the management of DM must also include a holistic approach that integrates nutrition and pharmaceuticals into the functional aspects of the life of individuals with DM or those at risk.

10. Treatment and management of diabetic cardiomyopathy

The flow diagram in **Figure 5** illustrates some interventions to treat and manage diabetic cardiomyopathy with the help of counseling for compliance, depression, and personal care. The standards in the treatment of diabetic cardiomyopathy are related to lifestyle modification, euglycemia, and mitigation of predisposing factors for cardiovascular diseases. Smoking cessation and alcohol consumption, healthy eating habits by decreasing carbohydrates and sugar consumption, reduction in body weight by eating a moderate amount daily, and daily aerobic exercise are the cornerstones in terms of lifestyle change (**Figure 5**).

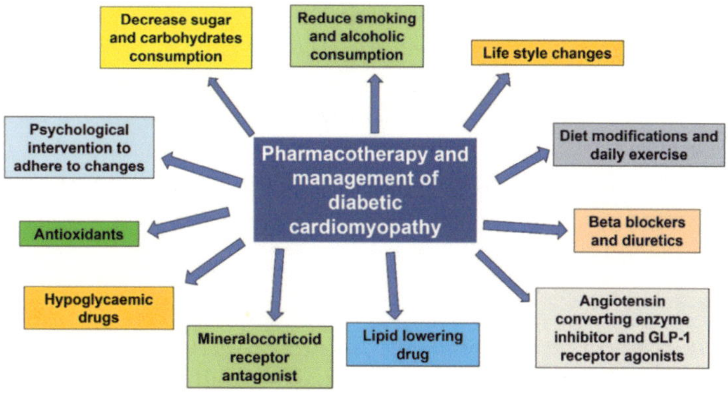

Figure 5.
A flow chart illustrating the interventions to manage and treat diabetic cardiomyopathy. GLP-1 = Glucagon-like-peptide-1.

10.1 Hypoglycemic agents

Several anti-diabetic drugs such as sulfonylureas, biguanides, inhibitors of α-glucosidase, thiazolidinediones, meglitinides, agonists of GLP-1 receptor, amylin analogs, and SGLT inhibitors are currently available for treating diabetes. These hypoglycemic agents can reduce blood glucose and HbA1c levels and enhance the well-being and the living standard of diabetic patients [70–74].

10.1.1 Sulfonylureas (SU)

Although some studies have shown that SU, when used alone, may elevate the risk of cardiovascular conditions, [75] a large clinical trial (CAROLINA Trial), conducted over 6 years, showed that the newer generation of SU (glimepiride) reduces the risk of major adverse cardiac events.

10.1.2 Biguanides

Several studies have shown that metformin can protect the heart, especially in DM patients. One study (UKPDS 34) reported that metformin mitigated MI in DM patients by almost 33%. Metformin can also alleviate the risk associated with MI, SCD, angina pectoris, and peripheral vascular disease by up to 30% in people suffering from DM because it can prevent inflammation and OS of the myocardium, and enhance microcirculation in the myocardial compartment of the heart [74, 76, 77].

10.1.3 α-glucosidase inhibitors

The beneficial effect of acarbose (an α-glucosidase inhibitor) in managing diabetic cardiomyopathy is controversial. Some studies (STOP-NIDDM multicenter, The meta-analysis of Risk Improvement under the use of Acarbose study) indicated that this α-glucosidase inhibitor can reduce MI, hypertension, and other cardiovascular risks by up to 34–64% [78, 79]. These observations contrasted those reported by the Acarbose Cardiovascular Evaluation Trial (ACET) on more than 6500 patients. ACET conducted in 176 centers showed that acarbose has no major beneficial effect on the heart [80].

10.1.4 Thiazolidinedione

The role of rosiglitazone and pioglitazone in the myocardium of the diabetic patient is controversial. Some reports (DREAM trial) have shown that these medications can cause HF [3, 81]. Although some reports have shown that this class of drugs can reduce stroke and MI [82], the consensus is that this group of anti-diabetic drugs can cause HF [83].

10.1.5 Meglitinides

Meglitinides have no marked effect on diabetic cardiomyopathy and have been reported to be subordinate to dipeptidyl peptidase-4 inhibitors, sodium-glucose co-transporter-2 inhibitors, and antagonists of GLP-1 receptors regarding the pharmacotherapy of cardiovascular conditions in DM patients [84, 85].

10.1.6 Dipeptidyl peptidase 4 inhibitors (DPP4i)

Several drugs such as vildagliptin, sitagliptin, denagliptin, and saxagliptin belong to the DPP4i class of drugs. Reports (CARMELINA, EXAMINE, TECOS) have shown that DPP4 inhibitors have no major effect on the heart and may even cause HF [86–89].

10.1.7 GLP-1 receptor agonists

Large clinical trials such as REWIND, HARMONY, PIONEER-6 reported that agonists of GLP-1 receptors curtail the risk for MI and the rate at which patients are hospitalized for heart HF [90].

10.1.8 SGLT inhibitors

SGLT2i displays a strong and significant reduction in cardiovascular events (MI, HF, stroke, hypertensive HF, and the rate of hospital stay for HF) in DM patients. This indicates that SGLT2i is non-hazardous and beneficial in DM patients and those with diabetes-induced cardiomyopathy [91, 92].

11. Structural treatment of the disease of coronary artery

Coronary artery lesions significantly contribute to the development, progression, and severity of DCM. One of the most important and recurring pathological lesions is atherosclerotic plaque. These plaques narrow the coronary artery lumen, which prevents adequate blood flow to the heart. Coronary artery stenosis may be so severe that revascularization may be needed to restore the perfusion of the myocardium.

In addition to treating the underlying DM and intensive medical therapy, currently, there are three major approaches to restoring the patency of a blocked or narrowed coronary artery. They include: a) graft bypass for coronary artery (CABG), or b) targeted vessel revascularization or PCI. PCI may employ either stents that elute drugs (DES) or naked metal stents. All of these procedures attempt to restore the function of coronary arteries and prevent stenosis and cardiovascular events.

DOI: http://dx.doi.org/10.5772/intechopen.1006679

In addition, it is also crucial to keep healthy nutrition, have a healthy total body weight and good lipid levels, achieve normal blood pressure and glucose levels, be active physically, and abstain from tobacco smoking [55, 93–98].

11.1 Which coronary artery restoration therapy is better?

While the use of medical treatment (anti-platelet, statins) and lifestyle changes (maintenance of healthy body weight, diet, good lipid profile, healthy blood pressure, and glucose concentrations, being active physically, and abstaining from tobacco smoking) is well agreed by all experts as being beneficial to patients with CAD, the restoration of the patency of coronary arteries is controversial. In a recent review comparing CABG with PCI, most experts believe that CABG is superior to PCI when restoring multiple coronary artery blockades. This is because CABG has a lower death rate and saves the patient from repeated revascularization compared to PCI, especially in patients with DM [55, 98].

Regarding PCI, drug-eluting stents are better than naked metal or balloon stents because of their ability to release medication, especially in DM patients. Patients with DES are unlikely to have recurring stenosis of the coronary artery when compared to those with balloon or bare metal stents [55].

12. What is new in the treatment of DCM?

12.1 Weight loss medications

Over the past few years, a new group of hypoglycemic medications, like antagonists to GLP-1 receptor (GLP-1 RA), have been utilized to treat overweight and obesity. These drugs are usually administered subcutaneously, however, oral formulations are also available for some classes of this medication. Many GLP-1R agonists (dulaglutide, exenatide, semaglutide) have now been manufactured for treating DM patients. Of these drugs, semaglutide has proved to be very effective in weight reduction. Semaglutide at a dose of 0.25 to 0.5 mg (sc; per os) per week can make significant reduction in total body weight. Millions of people worldwide now use semaglutide (Wegovy, Ozempic) for weight loss. In one study, semaglutide was able to induce a reduction of up to 15.8% of total body weight in 68 weeks [68, 69]. Despite the dramatic success of semaglutide in reducing body weight, the long-term adverse consequences of this "magic" drug are yet to be determined.

In an evaluation of RCTs of a large cohort of patients suffering from heart failure, GLP-1RA caused a significant improvement in cardiac function [99].

Consensus statements from several professional organizations, including the ACC Expert Consensus Panel on Novel Therapies for DM, EASD, ESC Guidelines on Diabetes, ACC/AHA on Primary Prevention of Cardiovascular Guidelines, and ADA, have suggested that GLP-1RA should be included as an "add-on" to the treatment of DCM [100]. Large RTCs have also pointed to the fact that GLP-1RAs markedly reduced cardiovascular outcomes in DM patients [70]. The rationale behind this consensus statement is that GLP-1RA can reduce obesity, insulin resistance, and inflammatory reactions [68], which predispose DM patients to developing DCM.

12.2 Sodium-glucose cotransporter-2 inhibitors (SGLT2i)

Several reports have shown that SGLT2i when given alone or with GLP-1RA possesses a strong cardio-protective effect, especially in DM patients. In many RCTs, including CREDENCE, EMPA-REG, and CANVAS, it was reported that SGLT2i significantly reduces fatal cardiovascular events and the rate of hospital visits due to HF [70, 101, 102]. The EMPEROR-Reduced RCT and VERTIS, which reviewed more than 10, 000 patients, reported that SGLT2i markedly mitigated the degree of severity of T2-DM-induced cardiovascular diseases [98, 103]. SGLT2i can alleviate the signs and symptoms of DCM because they improve microcirculation and the function of mitochondria. They also reduce the degree of cardiac fibrosis, oxidative stress, and ER stress [104].

13. Consensus in the management of diabetes-induced cardiomyopathy

The ADA and the EASD have recommended guidelines for the treatment of DM patients with cardiovascular diseases. In addition to PE, the first drug of choice should be metformin. The second recommended stage of treatment is a combination of metformin and GLP-1 R agonists. Other classes of drugs may be added in more severe cases of DCM [105].

14. Disability and quality of life (QoL) in DCM

DCM is a leading trigger of disability, along with a marked loss in quality of life. People with DM and DCM have a heightened risk of morbidity, severe loss of physical activity and function, including the incapability to perform daily tasks, as well as experiencing sexual and erectile dysfunctions. The estimated loss of activity could be as high as 80% of total capacity [106].

15. Ultrastructural changes in the diabetic heart

Diabetes mellitus (DM) causes severe morphological changes to the ultrastructure of the heart. The longer the duration of DM, the more destructive and drastic the alterations become. Nearly all of the cytoplasmic organelles are damaged by the impact of DM [15, 16, 107]. The mitochondria are swollen and turn into casts of organelles in severe cases. In addition, the myofibrils of the myocardium undergo marked degeneration with loss or thinning of structure. The discs of Eberth also suffer immense degeneration, resulting in loose contact between two adjacent cardiomyocytes (**Figure 6**).

16. Conclusion

In summary, the cellular events illustrated in **Figure 6** reveal how diabetes, if diagnosed late or left untreated, can induce heart disease such as cardiomyopathy. These pathophysiological processes are due to several metabolic, ultrastructural, and physiological changes in the myocardial layer of the heart. Recent research studies

DOI: http://dx.doi.org/10.5772/intechopen.1006679

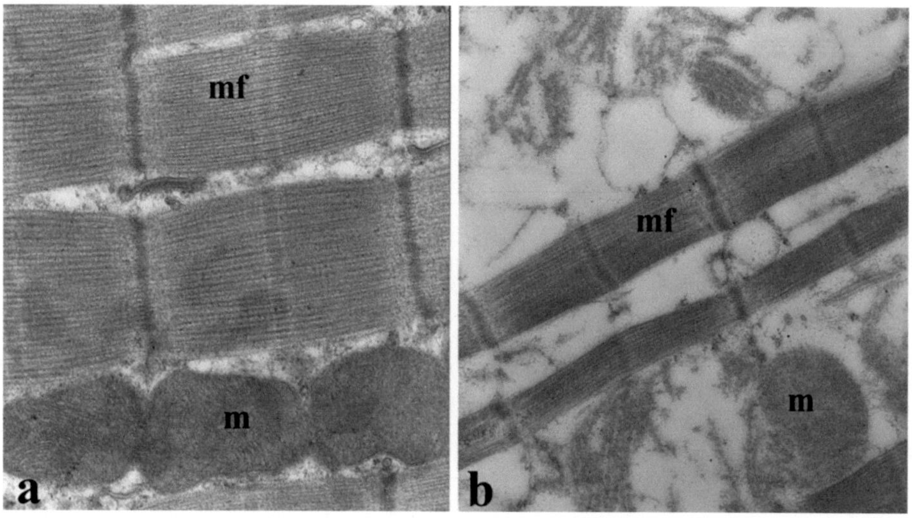

Figure 6.
TEM images of the myocardium of (a) control Wistar rat heart and (b) diabetic Wistar rat heart. Note the thinness of myofibrils and loss of mitochondria in diabetic hearts. Magnification: X27,500. TEM—Transmission electron microscope.

have helped significantly in understanding the pathophysiology of cardiac muscles, fibrosis infiltration, remodeling, derangement in cellular calcium homeostasis and contractile proteins, involvement of signature proteins and biomarkers and mediators, and physiological changes within the heart during DM. Further research on fatty acid metabolism, glucotoxicity, protein acetylation, and roles of potential biochemical markers for diabetic myocardiopathy including galectin-3 is required. As such, further studies are very important to comprehend the precise subcellular, cellular, and signaling cascades that take part in the initiation and progression of DCM. Furthermore, people must alter their lifestyle habits via diet modification by consuming lesser amount of carbohydrates and sugar but more green vegetables, participate in daily exercise, maintaining the correct basal metabolic index, adhere to medicine intake, and moreover, seek psychological intervention to adhere to these changes. In addition, there is an urgent need for further studies of the illness process and the discovery of more reliable clinical biomarkers of the disease. Moreover, to reduce mortality among diabetic patients, clinical practitioners must identify diabetic cardiomyopathy at an early stage and begin treatment.

Conflict of interest

The authors declared no conflict of interest.

Author details

Ernest A. Adeghate[1*], Sahar Mohsin[1], Ahmed Bin Amar[1], Suhail AlAmry[1], Mariam AlOtaiba[1], Omobola Awosika Oyeleye[2] and Jaipaul Singh[3]

1 Department of Human Anatomy, College of Medicine and Health Sciences, United Arab Emirates University, Al Ain, UAE

2 Cizik School of Nursing, University of Texas, Houston, Texas, USA

3 School of Pharmacy and Biomedical Sciences, University of Central Lancashire, Preston, England, UK

*Address all correspondence to: eadeghate@uaeu.ac.ae

References

[1] IDF Diabetes Atlas. International Diabetes Federation Diabetes Atlas. 10th ed. Brussels, Belgium: International Diabetes Federation; 2021

[2] American Diabetes Association Professional Practice Committee. Diabetes Care. 2024;**47**(Suppl 1):S20

[3] Mahgoub MO, Ali II, Adeghate JO, Tekes K, Kalász H, Adeghate EA. An update on the molecular and cellular basis of pharmacotherapy in type 2 diabetes mellitus. International Journal of Molecular Sciences. 2023;**24**(11):Article 9328

[4] Chatterjee S, Khunti K, Davies MJ. Type 2 diabetes. Lancet. 2017;**389**:2239-2251

[5] Good to Know. Race and type 2 diabetes. Clinical Diabetes. 2020;**38**(4):403-404. DOI: 10.2337/cd20-pe04

[6] Sattar N, Gill JMR. Type 2 diabetes in migrant south Asians: Mechanisms, mitigation, and management. The Lancet Diabetes and Endocrinology. 2015;**3**:1004-1016

[7] Yeo JL, Brady EM, McCann GP, Gulsin GS. Sex and ethnic differences in the cardiovascular complications of type 2 diabetes. Ther. Advances in Endocrinology and Metabolism. 2021;**12**:20420188211034297

[8] Adeghate E, Schattner P, Dunn E. An update on the Etiology and epidemiology of diabetes mellitus. Annals of the New York Academy of Sciences. 2006;**1084**:1-29

[9] Athithan L, Gulsin GS, , McCann GP, Levelt I. Diabetic cardiomyopathy: Pathophysiology, theories, and evidence to date. World Journal of Diabetes. 2019;**10**(10):490-510

[10] D' Souza A, Howarth CF, Yanni J, Dobrzynski H, Boyett MN, Adeghate E, et al. Chronic effect of mild hyperglycinemia on left ventricle transcriptional profile and structural remodeling in the spontaneously type 2 Goto-Kakizaki rat. Heart Failure Review. 2014;**19**:65-74. DOI: 10.1007/s10741-013-9376-9

[11] Rupee S, Rupe K, Singh RB, Hanoman C, Smail M, Singh J. Diabetes-induced chronic heart failure is due to defects in calcium transporting and regulatory contractile proteins: Cellular and molecular evidence. Heart Failure Review. 2022;**28**(3):627-644

[12] Zhang Y, Yang Z, Yani J, Qureshi MA, Logantha SJ, Kassab S, et al. Electrical conduction system remodelling in Streptozotocin-induced diabetes mellitus rat heart. Frontiers in Physiology. 2019;**10**:Article 826

[13] Lemasters JJ, DiGuiseppi NAL, Herman B. Blebbing, free Ca2+ and mitochondrial membrane potential preceding cell death in hepatocytes. Nature. 1987;**325**(6099):78-81

[14] Alomar FA, Al-Rubaish A, Al-Muhanna F, Al-Ali AA, McMillan JE, Singh J, et al. Adeno-associated viral transfer of glyoxalase-1 blunts carbonyl and oxidative stress in heart of type 1 diabetic rats. Antioxidants. 2020;**9**(7):Article 592 (22 pages). DOI: 10.3390/antiox9070592

[15] Adeghate E, Singh J. Structural changes in the myocardium during diabetes-induced cardiomyopathy.

Heart Failure Reviews. 2014;**19**(1):15-23. DOI: 10.1007/s10741-013-9388-5

[16] Adeghate E. Molecular and cellular basis of the aetiology and management of diabetic cardiomyopathy: A short review. Molecular and Cellular Biochemistry. 2004;**261**(1-2):187-191. DOI: 10.1023/b:mcbi.0000028755.86521.11

[17] Knowlton AA, Chen L, Malik ZA. Heart failure and mitochondrial dysfunction: The role of mitochondrial fission/fusion abnormalities and new therapeutic strategies. Journal of Cardiovascular Pharmacology. 2014;**63**(3):196-206

[18] De- Geest B, Mishra M. Role of oxidative stress in diabetic cardiomyopathy. Antioxidant. 2022;**11**(4):Article 784

[19] Lotfy M, Adeghate J, Kalasz H, Singh J, Adeghate E. Chronic complications of diabetes mellitus: A mini review. Current Diabetes Reviews. 2017;**13**(1):3-10. DOI: 10.2174/1573399812666151016101622

[20] Mongirdienė A, Skrodenis L, Varoneckaitė L, Mierkytė G, Gerulis J. Reactive oxygen species induced pathways in heart failure pathogenesis and potential therapeutic strategies. Biomedicine. 2022;**10**:602. DOI: 10.3390/biomedicines10030602

[21] Deanfield JE, Halcox JP, Rabelink TJ. Endothelial function and dysfunction: Testing and clinical relevance. Circulation. 2007;**115**:1285-1295

[22] Mironov AA, Mironov A, Sanavio B, Krol S, Beznoussenko GV. Intracellular membrane transport in vascular endothelial cells. International Journal of Molecular Sciences. 2023;**24**: Article 5791

[23] Deanfield JE, Halcox JP, Rabelink JJ. Endothelial function and dysfunction: Testing and clinical relevance. Circulation. 2007;**115**:1285-1296

[24] Avogaro A, Albiero M, Menegazzo L, de-Krewzenberg S, Fadini GP. Endothelial dysfunction in diabetes. Diabetes Care. 2011;**34**(Supple 2):S285-S290

[25] D'Souza A, Wang Y, Anderson C, et al. A circadian clock in the sinus node mediates day-night rhythms in Hcn4 and heart rate. Heart Rhythm. 2021;**18**(5):801-810

[26] Chang JL, Lee CJ, Suh K, You HU, Kim DH. Molecular properties of excitation-contraction coupling proteins in infant and adult human heart tissues. Molecules and Cells. 2005;**20**(1):51-56

[27] Widmaier EP, Raff H, Strang KT. Cardiac Muscle. In: Widmaier EP, Raff H, Strang KT, editors. Vander's Human Physiology - the Mechanisms of Body Function. 13th ed. New York: McGraw-Hill; 2014. pp. 292-294

[28] Labunde RE. Cardiac Excitation-Contraction Coupling. 2017. Available from: https://www.cvphysiology.com/Cardiac%20Function/CF022

[29] Berdowska E, Matusiewicz M, Feka I. Methylglyoxal in Cardiometabolic disorders: Routes leading to pathology counterbalanced by treatment strategies. Molecules. 2023;**28**(3):Article 7742

[30] Nigro C, Leone A, Fiory F, Prevenzano I, Nicolò A, Mirra P, et al. Dicarbonyl stress at the crossroads of healthy and unhealthy aging. Cells. 2019;**8**:Article 749

[31] Stratmann B. Dicarbonyl stress in diabetic vascular disease. International

Journal of Molecular Sciences. 2022;**23**:Article 6186

[32] Kosmicheskaya OV, Novikova NN, Topunov AF. Carbonyl stress in red blood cells and haemoglobin. Antioxidants. 2021;**10**:Article 253

[33] Tian C, Alomar F, More CJ, Shoa CH, Kutty S, Singh J, et al. Reactive carbonyl species and their roles in sarcoplasmic reticulum Ca2+ signaling in the diabetic heart. Heart Failure Reviews. 2016;**19**(1):101-112

[34] Azevedo PS, Polegato BF, Minicucci MF, Paiva SA, Zornoff LA. Cardiac remodelling: Concepts, clinical impact, pathophysiological mechanisms, and pharmacologic treatment. Arquivos Brasileiros de Cardiologia. 2016;**106**(1):62-69. DOI: 10.5935/abc.20160005

[35] Gregg EW, Sattar N, Ali MK. The changing face of diabetes complications. The Lancet Diabetes and Endocrinology. 2016;**4**:537-547

[36] Malhotra A, Lopez MC, Nakouzi A. Troponin subunits contribute to altered myosin ATPase activity in diabetic cardiomyopathy. Molecular and Cellular Biochemistry. 1995;**151**(2):165-172

[37] Hsueh WA, Wyne K. Renin-angiotensin-aldosterone system in diabetes and hypertension. Journal of Clinical Hypertension (Greenwich, Conn.). 2011;**13**(4):224-237. DOI: 10.1111/j.1751-7176.2011.00449.x

[38] Jia G, DeMarco VG, Sowers JR. Insulin resistance and hyperinsulinemia in diabetic cardiomyopathy. Nature Reviews. Endocrinology. 2016;**12**:144-153

[39] Mariappan N, Elks CM, Sriramula S, Guggilam A, Liu Z, Borkhsenious O, et al. NF-kappaB-induced oxidative stress contributes to mitochondrial and cardiac dysfunction in type II diabetes. Cardiovascular Research. 2010;**85**:473-483

[40] Chen J, Qin H, Hao J, Wang Q, Chen S, Yang G, et al. Cardiac-specific overexpression of CREM-IbΔC-X via CRISPR/Cas9 in mice presents a new model of atrial cardiomyopathy with spontaneous atrial fibrillation. Translational Research: The Journal of Laboratory and Clinical Medicine. 2024;**267**:54-66. DOI: 10.1016/j.trsl.2024.01.001

[41] Zhang K, Yuan Z, Wang S, Zhao S, Cui H, Lai Y. The abnormalities of free fatty acid metabolism in patients with hypertrophic cardiomyopathy, a single-center retrospective observational study. BMC Cardiovascular Disorders. 2024;**24**(1):312. DOI: 10.1186/s12872-024-03925-9

[42] Mahmoud LM, Mageed AAAA, Saadallah JM, Youssef MF, Rashed LA, Ammar HI. Interleukin 1β receptor blocker (Anakinra) and regenerative stem cell therapy: Two novel approaches effectively ameliorating diabetic cardiomyopathy. Naunyn-Schmiedeberg's Archives of Pharmacology. Advance online publication. 2024. DOI: 10.1007/s00210-024-03152-1

[43] Pacher P, Szabó C. Role of poly(ADP-ribose) polymerase 1 (PARP-1) in cardiovascular diseases: The therapeutic potential of PARP inhibitors. Cardiovascular Drug Reviews. 2007;**25**(3):235-260. DOI: 10.1111/j.1527-3466.2007.00018.x

[44] Yao X, Huang X, Chen J, Lin W, Tian J. Roles of non-coding RNA in diabetic cardiomyopathy. Cardiovascular Diabetology. 2024;**23**(1):227. DOI: 10.1186/s12933-024-02252-9

[45] Zuo G, Ren X, Qian X, Ye P, Luo J, Gao X, et al. Inhibition of JNK and p38 MAPK-mediated inflammation and apoptosis by ivabradine improves cardiac function in streptozotocin-induced diabetic cardiomyopathy. Journal of Cellular Physiology. 2019;**234**(2):1925-1936. DOI: 10.1002/jcp.27070

[46] Jia G, Hill MA, Sowers JR. Diabetic cardiomyopathy: An update of mechanisms contributing to this clinical entity. Circulation Research. 2018;**122**(4):624-638. DOI: 10.1161/CIRCRESAHA.117.311586

[47] de Paula AVL, Dykstra GM, da Rocha RB, Magalhães AT, da Silva BAK, Cardoso VS. The association of diabetic peripheral neuropathy with cardiac autonomic neuropathy in individuals with diabetes mellitus: A systematic review. Journal of Diabetes and its Complications. 2024;**38**(8):108802. DOI: 10.1016/j.jdiacomp.2024.108802

[48] Grundy S, Becker D, Clark LT, Cooper RS, Denke MA, Howard J, et al. Detection, evaluation, and treatment of high blood cholesterol in adults (adult treatment panel III). Circulation – Hagerstown. 2002;**106**:3143

[49] Newman AB, Siscovick DS, Manolio TA, Polak J, Fried LP, Borhani NO, et al. Ankle-arm index as a marker of atherosclerosis in the cardiovascular health study. Cardiovascular heart study (CHS) collaborative research group. Circulation. 1993;**88**(3):837-845

[50] Suzuki LA, Poot M, Gerrity RG, Bornfeldt KE. Diabetes accelerates smooth muscle accumulation in lesions of atherosclerosis: Lack of direct growth-promoting effects of high glucose levels. Diabetes. 2001;**50**(4):851-860

[51] Williams SB, Cusco JA, Roddy MA, Johnstone MT, Creager MA. Impaired nitric oxide-mediated vasodilation in patients with non-insulin-dependent diabetes mellitus. Journal of the American College of Cardiology. 1996;**27**(3):567-574

[52] Vinik AI, Erbas T, Park TS, Nolan R, Pittenger GL. Platelet dysfunction in type 2 diabetes. Diabetes Care. 2001;**24**(8):1476-1485

[53] Moreno PR, Murcia AM, Palacios IF, Leon MN, Bernardi VH, Fuster V, et al. Coronary composition and macrophage infiltration in atherectomy specimens from patients with diabetes mellitus. Circulation. 2000;**102**(18):2180-2184

[54] Marfella R, D'Amico M, Esposito K, Baldi A, Di FC, Siniscalchi M, et al. The ubiquitin-proteasome system and inflammatory activity in diabetic atherosclerotic plaques: Effects of rosiglitazone treatment. Diabetes. 2006;**55**(3):622-632

[55] Al-Nozha MM, Ismail HM, Al Nozha OM. Coronary artery disease and diabetes mellitus. Journal of Taibah University Medical Sciences. 2016;**11**(4):330-338

[56] Al Jaberi S, Cohen A, Saeed Z, Ojha S, Singh J, Adeghate E. Obesity: Molecular mechanisms, epidemiology, complications and pharmacotherapy. In: Cellular and Biochemical Mechanisms of Obesity. Advances in Biochemistry in Health and Disease. Switzerland: Springer; 2021. pp. 249-266. ISBN 978-3-030-84762-3

[57] Pickup JC. Inflammation and activated innate immunity in the pathogenesis of type 2 diabetes. Diabetes Care. 2004;**27**(3):813-823

[58] Albitar O, D'Souza CM, Adeghate EA. Effects of lipoproteins on metabolic

health. Nutrients. 2024;**16**(13):2156. DOI: 10.3390/nu16132156

[59] Laakso M. Cardiovascular disease in type 2 diabetes from population to man to mechanisms: The Kelly West award lecture 2008. Diabetes Care. 2010;**33**(2):442-449

[60] Luna-Luna M, Cruz-Robles D, Ávila-Vanzzini N, Herrera-Alarcón V, Martínez-Reding J, Criales-Vera S, et al. Differential expression of osteopontin, and osteoprotegerin mRNA in epicardial adipose tissue between patients with severe coronary artery disease and aortic valvular stenosis: Association with HDL subclasses. Lipids in Health and Disease. 2017;**16**(1):156. DOI: 10.1186/s12944-017-0550-2

[61] Wang Z, Song HY, An MM, Zhu LL. Association of serum SPARC level with severity of coronary artery lesion in type 2 diabetic patients with coronary heart disease. International Journal of Clinical and Experimental Medicine. 2015;**8**(10):19290-19296

[62] Campbell AP. DASH eating plan: An eating pattern for diabetes management. Diabetes Spectrum: A Publication of the American Diabetes Association. 2017;**30**(2):76-81

[63] Franz MJ, MacLeod J, Evert A, Brown C, Gradwell E, Handu D, et al. Academy of nutrition and dietetics nutrition practice guideline for type 1 and type 2 diabetes in adults: Systematic review of evidence for medical nutrition therapy effectiveness and recommendations for integration into the nutrition care process. Journal of the Academy of Nutrition and Dietetics. 2017;**117**(10):1659-1679

[64] Knutson KL. Impact of sleep and sleep loss on glucose homeostasis and appetite regulation. Sleep Medicine Clinics. 2007;**2**(2):187-197. DOI: 10.1016/j.jsmc.2007.03.004

[65] Sharma K, Akre S, Chakole S, Wanjari MB. Stress-induced diabetes: A review. Cureus. 2022;**14**(9):e29142. DOI: 10.7759/cureus.29142)

[66] Bornemisza P, Suciu I. Effect of cigarette smoking on the blood glucose level in normal and diabetics. Médecine Interne. 1980;**18**(4):353-356

[67] Emanuele NV, Swade TF, Emanuele MA. Consequences of alcohol use in diabetics. Alcohol Health and Research World. 1998;**22**(3):211-219

[68] Adeghate EA. GLP-1 receptor agonists in the treatment of diabetic non-alcoholic steatohepatitis patients. Expert Opinion on Pharmacotherapy. 2024;**25**(3):223-232. DOI: 10.1080/14656566.2024.2328796

[69] Rubino DM, Greenway FL, Khalid U, O'Neil PM, Rosenstock J, Sørrig R, et al. STEP 8 Investigators. Effect of weekly subcutaneous Semaglutide vs daily Liraglutide on body weight in adults with overweight or obesity without diabetes: The STEP 8 randomized clinical Trial. JAMA. 2022;**327**(2):138-150

[70] Adeghate EA, Kalász H, Al Jaberi S, Adeghate J, Tekes K. Tackling type 2 diabetes-associated cardiovascular and renal comorbidities: A key challenge for drug development. Expert Opinion on Investigational Drugs. 2021;**30**(2):85-93. DOI: 10.1080/13543784.2021.1865914

[71] Adeghate E, Mohsin S, Adi F, Ahmed F, Yahya A, Kalász H, et al. An update of SGLT1 and SGLT2 inhibitors in early phase diabetes-type 2 clinical trials. Expert Opinion on Investigational Drugs. 2019;**28**(9):811-820. DOI: 10.1080/13543784.2019.1655539

[72] Lotfy M, Singh J, Kalász H, Tekes K, Adeghate E. Medicinal chemistry and applications of Incretins and DPP-4 inhibitors in the treatment of type 2 diabetes mellitus. Open Medicinal Chemistry Journal. 2011;**5**(Suppl 2):82-92. DOI: 10.2174/1874104501105010082

[73] Adeghate E, Kalász H. Amylin analogues in the treatment of diabetes mellitus: Medicinal chemistry and structural basis of its function. Open Medicinal Chemistry Journal. 2011;**5**(Suppl. 2):78-81. DOI: 10.2174/1874104501105010078

[74] Adeghate E, Kalasz H, Veress G, Tekes K. Medicinal chemistry of drugs used in diabetic cardiomyopathy. Current Medicinal Chemistry. 2010;**17**(6):517-551. DOI: 10.2174/092986710790416281

[75] Azoulay L, Suissa S. Sulfonylureas and the risks of cardiovascular events and death: A methodological meta-regression analysis of the observational studies. Diabetes Care. 2017;**40**:706-714

[76] Petrie JR, Rossing PR, Campbell IW. Metformin and cardiorenal outcomes in diabetes: A reappraisal. Diabetes, Obesity & Metabolism. 2020;**22**:904-915

[77] Holman RR, Paul SK, Bethel MA, et al. 10-year follow-up of intensive glucose control in type 2 diabetes. The New England Journal of Medicine. 2008;**359**:1577-1589

[78] Chiasson JL, Josse RG, Gomis R, et al. STOP-NIDDM trial research group. Acarbose treatment and the risk of cardiovascular disease and hypertension in patients with impaired glucose tolerance: The STOP-NIDDM trial. Journal of the American Medical Association. 2003;**290**:486-494

[79] Hanefeld M, Cagatay M, Petrowitsch T, et al. Acarbose reduces the risk for myocardial infarction in type 2 diabetic patients: Meta-analysis of seven long-term studies. European Heart Journal. 2004;**25**:10-16

[80] Holman RR, Coleman RL, Chan JCN. Effects of acarbose on cardiovascular and diabetes outcomes in patients with coronary heart disease and impaired glucose tolerance (ACE): A randomised, double-blind, placebo-controlled trial. The Lancet Diabetes and Endocrinology. 2017;**5**:877-886. ACE Study Group

[81] Dagenais GR, Gerstein HC, Trial DREAM, Investigators. Effects of ramipril and rosiglitazone on cardiovascular and renal outcomes in people with impaired glucose tolerance or impaired fasting glucose: Results of the diabetes REduction assessment with ramipril and rosiglitazone medication (DREAM) trial. Diabetes Care. 2008;**31**:1007-1014

[82] Zhou Y, Huang Y, Ji X, et al. Pioglitazone for the primary and secondary prevention of cardiovascular and renal outcomes in patients with or at high risk of type 2 diabetes mellitus: A meta-analysis. The Journal of Clinical Endocrinology and Metabolism. 2020;**105**(5):dgz252

[83] Lipscombe LL, Gomes T, Lévesque LE, Hux JE, Juurlink DN, Alter DA. Thiazolidinediones and cardiovascular outcomes in older patients with diabetes. Journal of the American Medical Association. 2007;**298**(22):2634-2643. DOI: 10.1001/jama.298.22.2634

[84] Holman RR, Haffner SM, McMurray JJ. Effect of nateglinide on the incidence of diabetes and cardiovascular events. NAVIGATOR study group. The New England Journal of Medicine. 2010;**362**(16):1463-1476

[85] O'Brien MJ, Karam SL, Wallia A, et al. Association of second-line

antidiabetic medications with cardiovascular events among insured adults with type 2 diabetes. JAMA Network Open. 2018;**1**:e186125

[86] McGuire DK, Alexander JH, Johansen OE, CARMELINA investigators. Linagliptin effects on heart failure and related outcomes in individuals with type 2 diabetes mellitus at high cardiovascular and renal risk in CARMELINA. Circulation. 2019;**139**:351-361

[87] Scirica BM, Bhatt DL, Braunwald E, et al. Saxagliptin and cardiovascular outcomes in patients with type 2 diabetes mellitus. The New England Journal of Medicine. 2013;**369**:1317-1326

[88] Furuhashi M, Sakuma I, Morimoto T, et al. Treatment with anagliptin, a DPP-4 inhibitor, decreases FABP4 concentration in patients with type 2 diabetes mellitus at a high risk for cardiovascular disease who are receiving statin therapy. Cardiovascular Diabetology. 2020;**19**(1):89

[89] Zhang Z, Chen X, Lu P, et al. Incretin-based agents in type 2 diabetic patients at cardiovascular risk: Compare the effect of GLP-1 agonists and DPP-4 inhibitors on cardiovascular and pancreatic outcomes. Cardiovascular Diabetology. 2017;**16**:31

[90] Giugliano D, Maiorino MI, Bellastella G, et al. GLP-1 receptor agonists for prevention of cardiorenal outcomes in type 2 diabetes: An updated meta-analysis including the REWIND and PIONEER 6 trials. Diabetes, Obesity & Metabolism. 2019;**21**:2576-2580

[91] Wilcox T, De Block C, Schwartzbard AZ, et al. Diabetic agents, from metformin to SGLT2 inhibitors and GLP1 receptor agonists: JACC focus seminar. Journal of the American College of Cardiology. 2020;**75**:1956-1974

[92] Mahaffey KW, Neal B, Perkovic V, et al. Canagliflozin for primary and secondary prevention of cardiovascular events: Results from the canvas program (canagliflozin cardiovascular assessment study). Circulation. 2018;**137**:323-334

[93] Frye RL, August P, Brooks MM, Hardison RM, Kelsey SF, MacGregor JM, et al. A randomized trial of therapies for type 2 diabetes and coronary artery disease. The New England Journal of Medicine. 2009;**360**(24):2503-2515

[94] Mehran R, Dangas GD, Kobayashi Y, Lansky AJ, Mintz GS, Aymong ED, et al. Short- and long-term results after multivessel stenting in diabetic patients. Journal of the American College of Cardiology. 2004;**43**(8):1348-1354

[95] West NE, Ruygrok PN, Disco CM, Webster MW, Lindeboom WK, O'Neill WW, et al. Clinical and angiographic predictors of restenosis after stent deployment in diabetic patients. Circulation. 2004;**109**(7):867-873

[96] Bangalore S, Kumar S, Fusaro M, Amoroso N, Kirtane AJ, Byrne RA, et al. Outcomes with various drug eluting or bare metal stents in patients with diabetes mellitus: Mixed treatment comparison analysis of 22,844 patient-years of follow-up from randomized trials. BMJ. 2012;**345**:e5170

[97] Milojevic M, Head SJ, Parasca CA, Serruys PW, Mohr FW, Morice MC, et al. Causes of death following PCI versus CABG in complex CAD: 5-year follow-up of SYNTAX. Journal of the American College of Cardiology. 2016;**67**(1):42-55

[98] Spadaccio C, Benedetto U. Coronary artery bypass grafting (CABG) vs. percutaneous coronary intervention (PCI) in the treatment of multivessel

coronary disease: Quo vadis? -a review of the evidences on coronary artery disease. Annals of Cardiothoracic Surgery. 2018;**7**(4):506-515. DOI: 10.21037/acs.2018.05.1

[99] Ternes C, Sirena E, Colares F, et al. GLP-1 receptor agonists rising role in heart failure management: A systematic review and meta-analysis. JACC. 2024;**83**(13_Supplement):391. DOI: 10.1016/S0735-1097(24)023817

[100] Khan MS, Fonarow GC, McGuire DK, Hernandez AF, et al. Glucagon-like peptide 1 receptor agonists and heart failure: The need for further evidence generation and practice guidelines optimization. Circulation; **142**(12):1205-1218. DOI: 10.1161/CIRCULATIONAHA.120.045888

[101] Zhou H. SGLT2 inhibitors: A novel player in the treatment and prevention of diabetic cardiomyopathy. Drug Design, Development and Therapy. 2020;**14**:4775-4788. DOI: 10.2147/DDDT.S269514

[102] Li N, Zhou H. SGLT2 inhibitors: A novel player in the treatment and prevention of diabetic cardiomyopathy. Drug Design, Development and Therapy. 2020;**14**:4775-4788. DOI: 10.2147/DDDT.S269514

[103] Cosentino F, Cannon CP, Cherney DZI, et al. Efficacy of ertugliflozin on heart failure-related events in patients with type 2 diabetes mellitus and established atherosclerotic cardiovascular disease: Results of the VERTIS CV trial. Circulation. 2020;**142**:2205-2215. Epub ahead of print

[104] Huang K, Luo X, Liao B, et al. Insights into SGLT2 inhibitor treatment of diabetic cardiomyopathy: Focus on the mechanisms. Cardiovascular Diabetology. 2023;**22**:86. DOI: 10.1186/s12933-023-01816-5

[105] Bashier A, Bin Hussain A, Abdelgadir E, Alawadi F, Sabbour H, Chilton R. Consensus recommendations for management of patients with type 2 diabetes mellitus and cardiovascular diseases. Diabetology and Metabolic Syndrome. 2019;**11**:80. DOI: 10.1186/s13098-019-0476-0.], 10.1186/s13098-019-0476-0.]

[106] Oyewole OO, Ale AO, Ogunlana MO, Gurayah T. Burden of disability in type 2 diabetes mellitus and the moderating effects of physical activity. World Journal of Clinical Cases. 2023;**11**(14):3128-3139. DOI: 10.12998/wjcc.v11.i14.3128.]

[107] Howarth FC, Qureshi MA, Lawrence P, Adeghate E. Chronic effects of streptozotocin-induced diabetes on the ultrastructure of rat ventricular and papillary muscle. Acta Diabetologica. 2000;**37**(3):119-124. DOI: 10.1007/s005920070013

Chapter 6

Left Ventricle Arrhythmogenic Cardiomyopathy in Canines and Felines

Guillermo Belerenian, Cristian Daniel Rodríguez, Víctor Castillo and Gustavo Abuin

Abstract

This chapter describes pathological, electrocardiographic, echocardiographic, and clinical findings of two cases, one in a canine and the other in a feline, which suggest the presence of Left Ventricle Arrhythmogenic Cardiomyopathy. It is considered to be of interest for comparative medicine. To the authors' knowledge, it's the first ever description of the pathology carried out in companion animals. The canine patient arrived at the clinic with arrhythmias. After 48 hours, he had a sudden death and the heart was studied, finding a partial replacement of the free wall and septum of the left ventricle with fatty tissue. The feline patient also had a sudden death, and the heart was studied, where transmural replacement of the myocardium from the free wall of the left ventricle was found, which was replaced by adipose tissue.

Keywords: arrhythmogenic cardiomyopathy, feline, canine, adipose replacement, arrhythmia

1. Introduction

Arrhythmogenic Cardiomyopathy is a genetic disease of the heart muscle characterized by the replacement of the myocardium with fibroadipose tissue [1]. The onset of the substitution begins in the epicardium and progresses over time toward the mesomyocardium. The disease was originally called Right Ventricle Arrhythmogenic Dysplasia because that was the phenotype which was first discovered. The new knowledge about it highlights a genotype-phenotype correlation, and the characterization of the myocardial tissue through cardiac magnetic resonance in the human species demonstrated the involvement of the left ventricle. Nowadays, it is called Arrhythmogenic Cardiomyopathy because it can involve both ventricles, or predominantly the right ventricle or predominantly the left ventricle.

In this chapter, we report two cases of left ventricle predominant Arrhythmogenic Cardiomyopathy in companion animals. The existing evidence suggests that it could be more prevalent in the Boxer and in the English Bulldog breeds, when speaking of canines, even though the authors found it in a Fila Brasilero dog [2]. This form of Arrhythmogenic Cardiomyopathy may resemble dilated cardiomyopathy or myocarditis, and it appears that there is a genetic basis for these two different phenotypes [3].

To summarize, nowadays we can find the right-predominant phenotype, the left-predominant phenotype, and the biventricular phenotypic variant of the disease [4].

2. Phenotype

Studies of anatomic pathology in human beings who presented right ventricle Arrhythmogenic Cardiomyopathy showed evidence of macroscopic and histological involvement of the left ventricle in up to 76% of the cases. It was affecting the free wall and the septum, most often regionally, and the most involved areas were the posteroseptal and posterolateral. The lesion was located in the outer layer, which had areas of replacement fibrosis or subepicardial fibrofatty change [5].

The phenotypic features of Left Ventricle Arrhythmogenic Cardiomyopathy in humans include electrocardiogram (ECG) abnormalities, such as low-amplitude Quality Rating System (QRS), in the limb's derivations or t-wave inversion or flattening in the inferolateral derivations, as well as ventricular arrhythmias with right bundle branch block morphology (a ventricular conduction disorder that can happen in any of the two ventricles), which denotes its origin at the left ventricle.

Echocardiogram (Echo) shows a normal or mildly depressed left ventricle's systolic function, without or with mild dilation. When performing a cardiac magnetic resonance imaging with contrast, fibrosis in the subepicardial layers at the inferior or inferolateral regions is evidenced. The subendocardial layer is conserved, so regional contractility may be at a normal state. Therefore, echocardiography is sometimes not as useful for diagnosis as magnetic resonance imaging (MRI), which is a limitation for animal cardiology since this diagnostic method is not so easily available in companion animals [6].

3. Genotype

In Arrhythmogenic Cardiomyopathy, most pathological mutations affect genes that encode proteins that are structural for the intercellular binding of myocytes. Among these proteins, the most found at a mutated state are: Plakophylin, Desmoplakin, Desmoglein, and Desmocollin. Rarer are those mutations affecting Alpha-T-Catenin and N-cadherin. Mutations were also found in nondesmosomic genes, such as Phospholamban, Mylamin, Desmin, Titin, and Lamina A and C.1. These latter mutations are also associated with dilated cardiomyopathy and, therefore, may have overlapping phenotypes [7]. There also exist mutations in transmembrane proteins, such as Transmembrane Protein 43 or the Transforming Growth Factor Beta-3 (TGF-β3).

Genotype-phenotype correlation studies on human medicine showed that the mutations in genes that synthesize proteins, such as Desmoplakin, Phospholamban, Filamin C, Lamina A and C, Desmin, and Transmembrane Protein 43, specifically affect the left ventricle primarily before affecting the right ventricle [8]; while the mutations of Plakophylin C, Desmoglein, Desmocollin, and Plakoglobin affect the right ventricle primarily. Phospholamban inhibits the calcium transport of adenosine phosphatase (ATPase) of the sarcoplasmic reticulum (SR), so mutations dysregulate calcium flow predisposing to arrhythmia and ventricular dysfunction. Phospholamban mutations were found in boxer dog family groups [9].

4. Diagnosis

In human medicine, the Padua criteria are used to diagnose and phenotypically categorize Arrhythmogenic Cardiomyopathy, using major and minor criteria for each method and for each region.

For predominantly right affectation (that's to say, when the right ventricle is predominantly affected), the major criteria by echocardiography are right ventricular morphofunctional anomalies, akinesia, dyskinesia or regional dilation of the right ventricle, and dilation or global systolic dysfunction of the right ventricle. And the minor criteria are regional right ventricle akinesia or aneurysm of the right ventricle free wall.

On the other hand, for predominantly left affectation, the major criteria are global systolic dysfunction of the left ventricle with depression of the shortening fraction, with or without dilation of the left ventricle; and a minor criterion would be left regional hypokinesia or akinesia of the free wall or septum.

The major criteria for cardiac magnetic resonance imaging for each sector are transmural anomalies that suggest a fibrous replacement of the myocardium in the septum or in the free wall, while the minor criteria would be very restricted fibrous replacement lesions, either in the septum or in the free wall [10]. Major and minor criteria are also applied with the use of the electrocardiogram as a diagnostic method. Respecting the repolarization abnormalities, a major criterion for the right ventricle would be inverted t-waves in the right precordial leads V1 V2 V3; and a major criterion for the left ventricle would be inverted waves in the left precordial leads V4 V5 V6, always in the absence of left bundle branch block. Minor criteria would be inverted t-waves in two precordial derivations for both ventricles.

About the depolarization anomalies, a major criterion would be the appearance of epsilon waves, which would be low-amplitude signals between the end of the QRS complex and the beginning of the t-wave in right precordial derivations from V1 to V3. In the left ventricle, a major criterion would also be the appearance of low QRS voltages lesser than 0.1 millivolt in the limb leads [11]. Another major criterion for the right-predominant condition is the emergence of frequent ventricular extrasystoles, greater than 500 in 24 hours, or a sustained or nonsustained ventricular tachycardia with left bundle branch block morphology. In the case of the left-predominant condition, it would be the same but with a sustained or nonsustained ventricular tachycardia with right bundle branch block morphology. A minor criterion for both ventricles would be ventricular extrasystoles minor to 500 in 24 hours. Lastly, genetic family history (whether there are known mutations for the disease in the family research) is important. In veterinary medicine, these criteria are not established [12].

The studies carried out on animals have been done mainly on canines from the Boxer and English Bulldog breeds, but they have not been able to establish any diagnostic criteria, although it is allowed to suspect the disease when a 24/48-hour rhythm Holter is done and more than 1000 premature ventricular complexes appear daily with morphology of left bundle branch block (in the case of suspected involvement of the right ventricle) and with morphology of right bundle branch block (if left ventricle involvement is suspected) [13]. It is also important to correlate it with echocardiographic changes, in addition to the criteria detailed above. If right ventricle Arrhythmogenic Cardiomyopathy is suspected, the right ventricular cavity may be dilated, the wall may be very thin, or there may also be regional or global motility alterations; the TAPSE (Tricuspid Annular Plane Systolic Excursion) and the right ventricle ejection fraction may be decreased. In the case of the left ventricle, ejection fraction, shortening fraction, and MAPSE (Mitral Annular Plane Systolic Excursion) may be decreased. There may also be regional or global motility alterations and the wall may be thinner, which is less frequent in canines.

In the case of felines, we will see that a wall of the left ventricle was found completely replaced by fat and it became thinner. Clinically, syncope or sudden death predominates. Alterations in biomarkers, such as ventricular natriuretic peptide and troponin, may appear [14].

5. Description of the canine case

A 2-year-old male Brazilian Fila canine with a history of syncope during exercise was presented to the cardiology clinic. On clinical examination, the auscultation revealed an irregular rhythm, and no murmurs were detected. The weight of the animal was 20 kg. The blood chemistry and hemogram parameters were within normal limits.

A six-lead electrocardiogram showed the presence of isolated premature ventricular complexes with right bundle branch block morphology. Then, the echocardiogram showed an increase in the diameter of the left ventricle diastole ending part (62 mm) normalized to body weight, with a shortening fraction of 41% and an ejection fraction of 71% (preserved). A 24-hour Holter monitoring was indicated, which was performed the next day, and a complete blood test was also indicated, the results of which were normal [15]. The patient remained at home during the Holter study. A three-channel study was performed, and the recording showed baseline sinus rhythm during 95% of the study time. The maximum heart rate was 231 beats per minute and the minimum was 54 beats. There were 11 episodes of supraventricular tachycardia lasting 3 seconds on average. A total of 93 complexes of ventricular origin were detected, approximately 50% of which were escape beats. All ventricular escape complexes had left bundle branch block morphology, while premature ventricular complexes had right bundle branch block morphology (**Figures 1** and 2). During the study, an increase in the QT interval was observed, corrected by Basset's formula (**Figure 3**). After 24 hours of performing the rhythm Holter, the patient died suddenly while performing physical activity. After the animal's death, authorization was obtained to perform the necropsy.

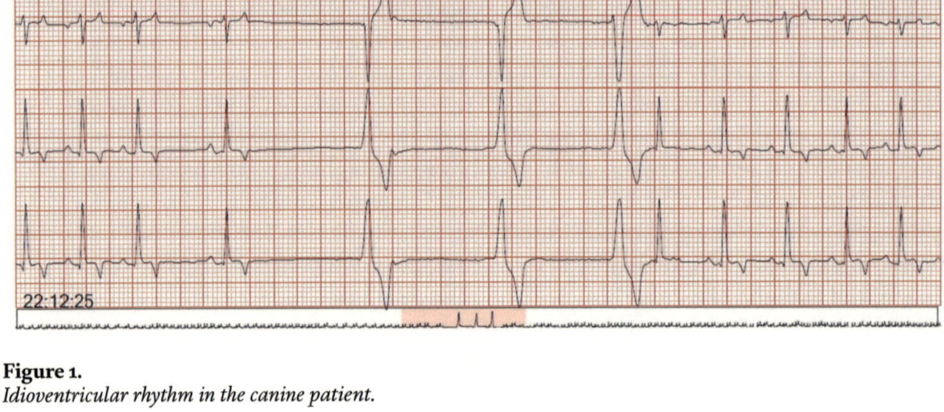

Figure 1.
Idioventricular rhythm in the canine patient.

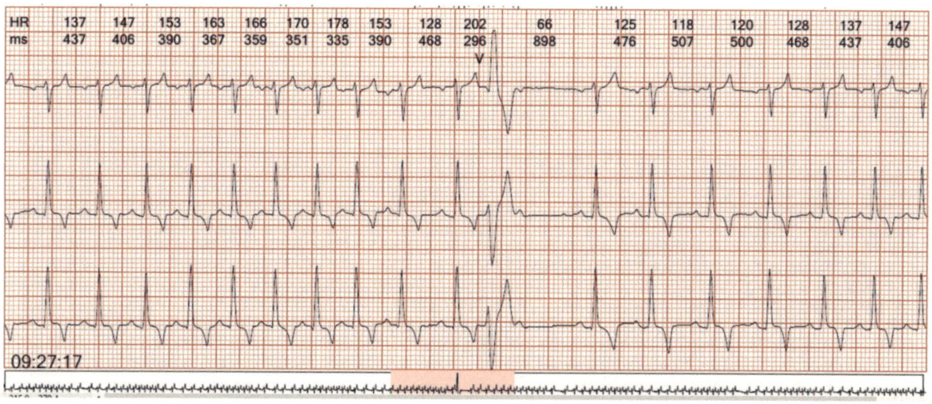

Figure 2.
Ventricular premature complexes with right bundle branch block morphology in the canine.

Fc	91	111	130	150	170	213	125
QT	0,2	0,2	0,2	0,2	0,2	0,2	0,22
rr	0,64	0,52	0,38	0,4	0,36	0,28	0,46
raíz de rr	0,8	0,72	0,61	0,63	0,6	0,52	0,67
QTc	0,25	0,27777778	0,32786885	0,38461538	0,38461538	0,38461538	0,32835821

Figure 3.
QT corrected by Basset's formula.

During the study, a clear cardiomegaly was evidenced, the weight of the heart was greater than 13 grams of cardiac tissue for every kilogram of body weight. No pulmonary edema, pleural effusion, or ascites were observed. The heart was exposed, preserved in 10% formaldehyde, and sent for study to the pathology service of the Hospital Santojani in the Ciudad Autónoma de Buenos Aires. Slices were made with hematoxylin–eosin staining, after including the paraffin samples. In the free wall of the left ventricle, a predominantly subepicardial fat replacement was observed and the septum on the left side was affected (**Figure 4**) [16]. The base of implantation of the papillary muscles was also affected, where replacement by adipose tissue was found (**Figure 5**). Perivascular fibrosis and replacement fibrosis also coexisted in some areas of the left ventricle, suggesting a lesion that led to necrosis and fibrosis. Myocardial wavy fibers were also found in both ventricles, and preserved myocardial muscle fibers were found within the fibrofat replacement islets (**Figures 6** and 7). This led to the finding of a suggestive left-predominant arrhythmogenic cardiomyopathy. There were no signs of congestive heart failure. No signs of myocarditis were observed. Fat replacement of up to 50% of the free wall was also found in some areas of the right ventricle, but this was very localized. There is a possibility that physical activity may have triggered the hot phase of the disease, and mechanical stress may have caused the decoupling of more myocytes, with the consequent secondary injury with predisposition to ventricular arrhythmias and sudden death [17].

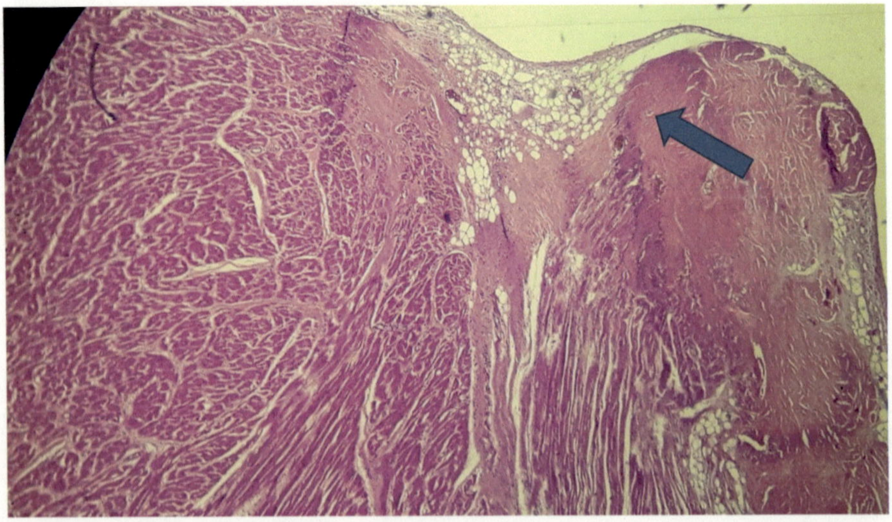

Figure 4.
Histopathological image of the interventricular septum with fat replacement. The arrow points to the fatty replacement area in the interventricular septum.

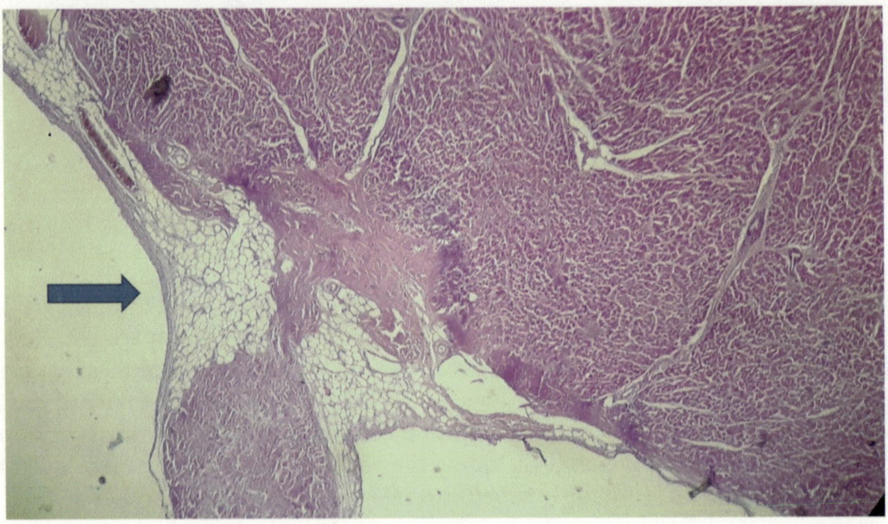

Figure 5.
Histopathological image. Staining with hematoxylin and eosin. Canine left ventricle. Papillary muscle base fat replacement. The arrow points to the fatty replacement at the papillary muscle implantation site.

6. Feline case description

A 3-year-old male European common cat was presented to the emergency room. It was neutered and had had syncope. Routine auscultation revealed an arrhythmia. An electrocardiogram was performed, in which ventricular tachycardia with right bundle branch block morphology was observed in the tachycardia beats (**Figure 8**). The blood analysis were within normal parameters.

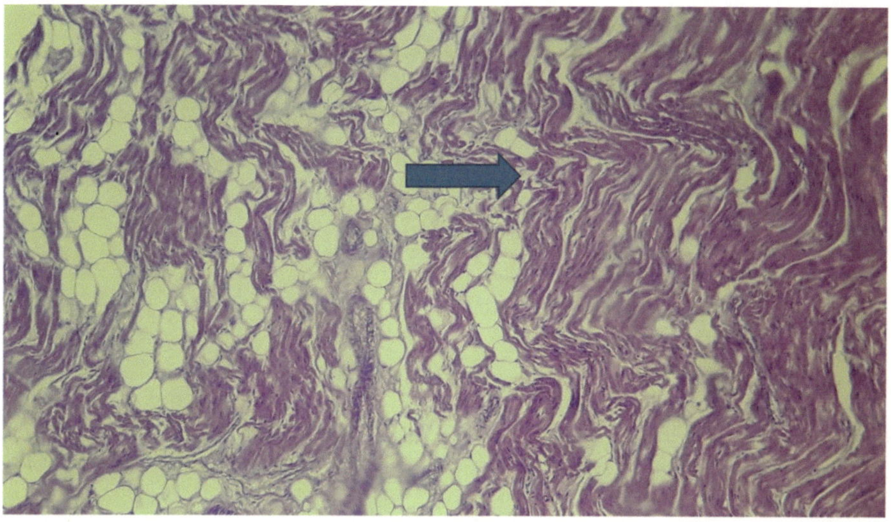

Figure 6.
The arrow points to the myocardial wavy fibers in areas of fat replacement.

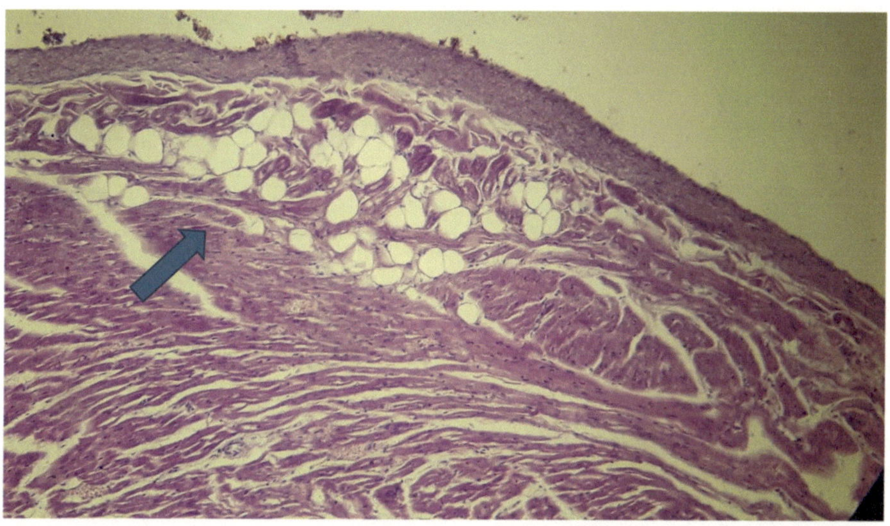

Figure 7.
The arrow points to the subepicardial fibrofatty replacement in the canine left ventricular wall.

The patient is scheduled the next day for an echocardiogram, but it faces a sudden death at home. Permission is obtained from the owners to perform the necropsy. The anterolateral free wall of the left ventricle was completely replaced by fat and there were no abnormalities in the epicardial coronary arteries that ran through the entire wall, even in the segment where the fat replacement was located. The histopathological study did not reveal coronary artery disease nor was there any thromboembolism or atheromatous plaques along the coronary artery branches that crossed the segment replaced by fat. However, a virtually total replacement of the free wall of the left ventricle was found, with very little subendocardial tissue preserved and the entire epicardium, subepicardium, and mesomyocardium replaced by fatty tissue (**Figure 9**). This also led to the suspicion that the arrhythmia originated in the left ventricle, given the morphology of the complexes and that the fatty replacement of that segment of the free wall of the left ventricle was the origin of the arrhythmia that produced the sudden death. In this case, the staining was also performed with hematoxylin–eosin (**Figures 10–12**).

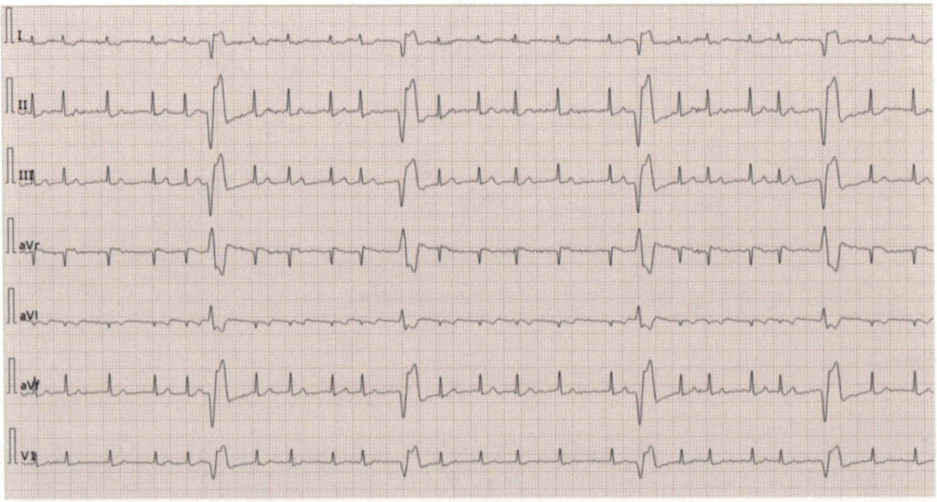

Figure 8.
Ventricular extrasystoles with right bundle branch block morphology in the feline patient.

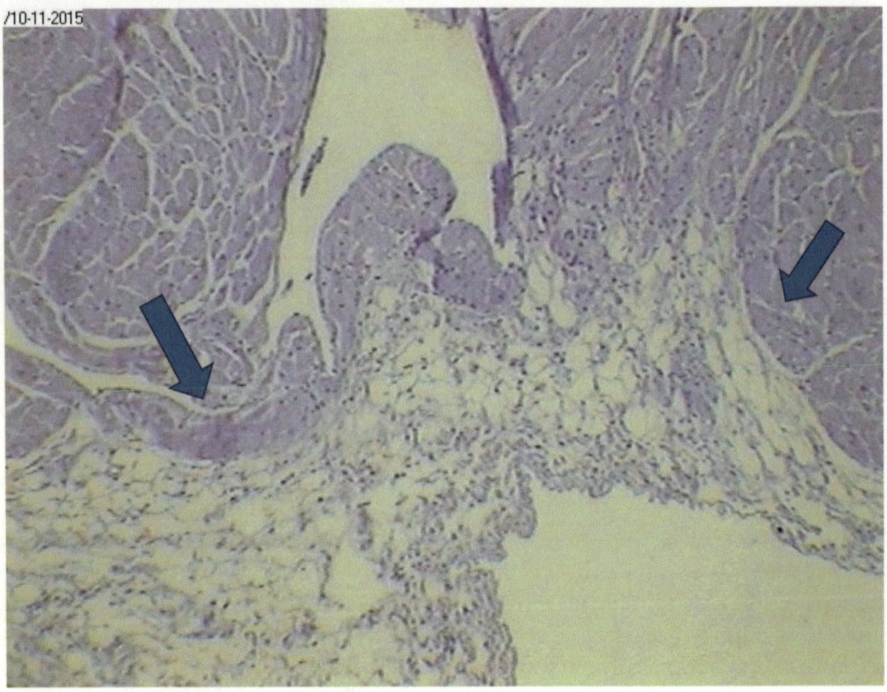

Figure 9.
Histopathological image of the feline patient. Fat replacement of the free wall of the left ventricle with preserved subendocardium. The arrow points to the fatty replacement in the epicardium.

To the knowledge of the authors, left ventricle Arrhythmogenic Cardiomyopathy in companion animals has not yet been described. It should be noted that in these two cases, there were no signs of heart failure prior to death, so it is estimated that death was due to arrhythmia [12].

7. Discussion

In the classic form of right ventricle Arrhythmogenic Dysplasia, now called Arrhythmogenic Heart Disease, the overall function of the left ventricle is usually not affected. The involvement of both ventricles usually occurs in the outer third of the

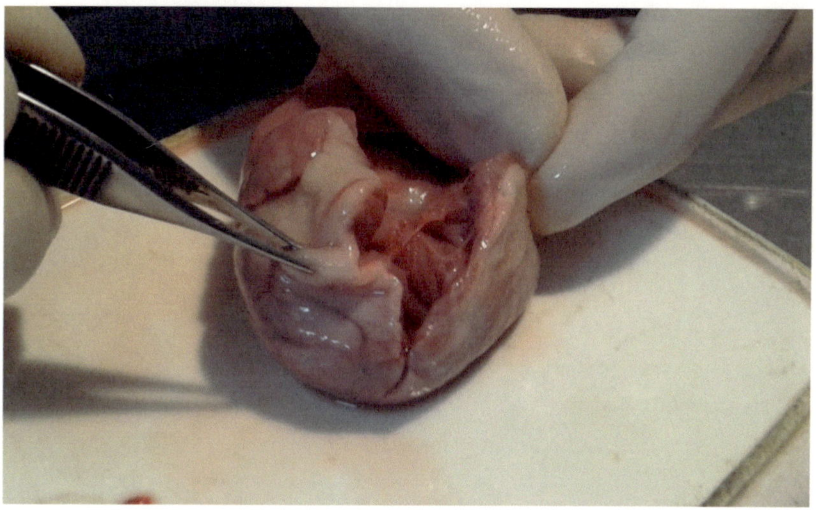

Figure 10.
The forceps take the free wall of the feline patient's left ventricle replaced by fat.

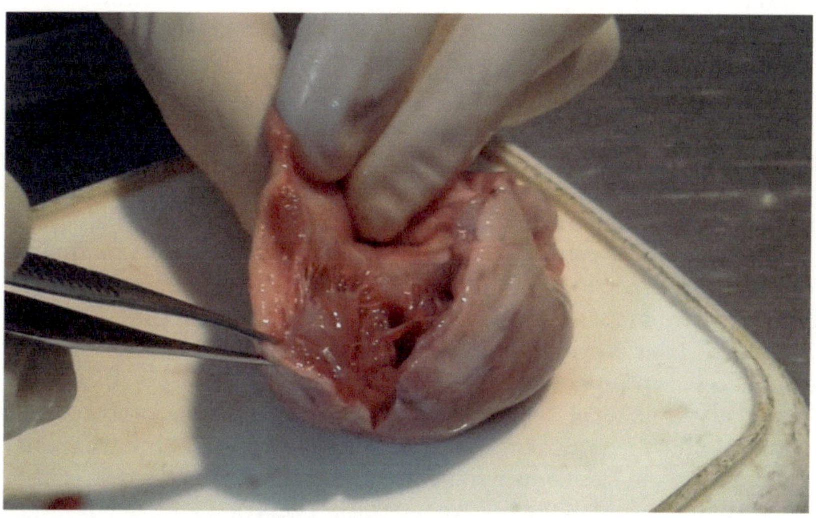

Figure 11.
Preserved myocardium is observed above below the fatty replacement of the ventricle wall.

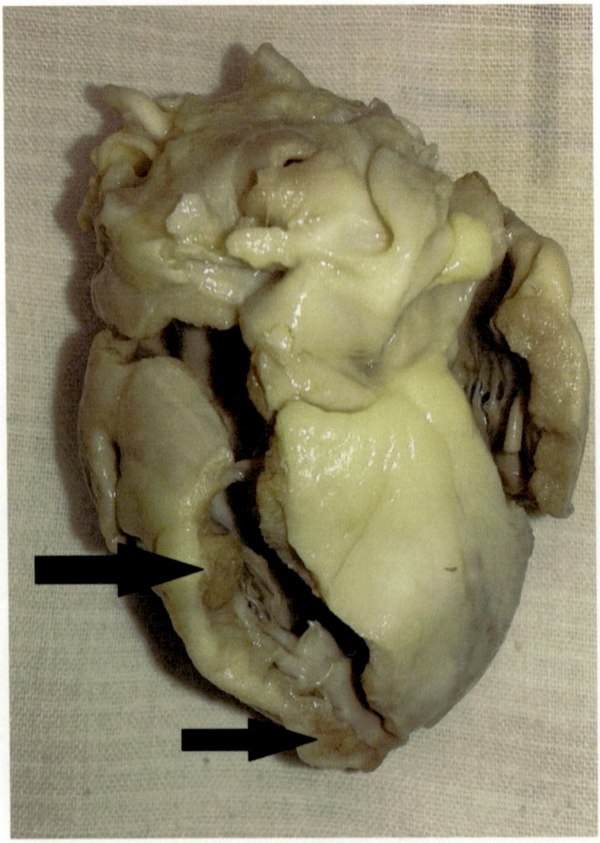

Figure 12.
Formaldehyde piece from the previous case. The arrows show the remnant of myocardium preserved in the free wall replaced by fat.

myocardium and, in general, on the right side of the interventricular septum. In the present canine case, the structural abnormalities found during the echocardiographic study corresponded to an increase in diastolic diameter, preserving the shortening fraction without evidence of alterations in the thickness of the free wall of the left ventricle or septum.

In the left dominant form of Arrhythmogenic Cardiomyopathy, the distribution of fibrosis usually predominates in the outer third, that's to say, in the epicardium and subepicardium, and progresses to the endocardium. This lesion may have a circumferential shape or may be patchy. The left form of Arrhythmogenic Cardiomyopathy may or may not be associated with dilation of the right ventricle. In the classic form of the disease, ventricular tachycardia with left bundle branch block morphology can be observed, while in the left ventricular form, ventricular tachycardia will present right bundle branch block morphology.

In human medicine reports of the left-predominant form, the interventricular septum was affected in more than 50%. These findings coincide with what was observed in the present canine case and with what was found in the feline, where the fat replacement took place in the free wall of the left ventricle [18]. On the other hand, the difference observed in the present case differs with respect to the biventricular form, because in this case there is right and left dilation, and in our canine and feline cases, the dilation was only on the left side. The right ventricle in both cases was normal. In human medicine, before the disease is in a highly advanced stage, it is difficult to differentiate the left form from the biventricular presentation. It's the same when distinguishing dilated cardiomyopathy of the left form from Arrhythmogenic Heart Disease, because the subepicardial distribution of the lesion must be taken into account, which is more frequent in the left form of the disease than in the dilated one [19].

Another differential feature that supports the diagnosis of the left dominant form over the dilated form is the presence of severe ventricular arrhythmia in the arrhythmogenic form, which is disproportionately high for the degree of systolic involvement of the left ventricle. The same happens with the appearance of congestive heart failure. That is a final event in Arrhythmogenic Cardiomyopathy, whereas in dilated cardiomyopathy, it is an initial event. Cases with classic Arrhythmogenic Heart Disease arrive with arrhythmia with normal left ventricular systolic function. Additionally, in predominantly right-sided Arrhythmogenic Cardiomyopathy, the left-sided septum is much less affected than the right-sided septum. In our canine case, septal involvement was a distinguishing feature to suspect a left form of the disease, while in our feline case the septum was preserved. Another differential diagnosis in the findings observed in this report is the ischemic heart disease.

When speaking of ischemic heart disease, fibrosis with subendocardial disposition is usually observed, which can be transmural after progressing. In our report of the canine case, there was an epicardial and midventricular lesion but without dysfunction or dilation of the left ventricle and without coronary involvement [20]. This also shows that, between the studies by imaging, the echocardiogram has low sensitivity to detect this type of lesion and it is very important to consider the use of magnetic resonance imaging (MRI) with gadolinium as contrast to further improve the diagnosis [21]. On the other hand, the mutations discovered (both in humans and animals) of the genes encoding desmosomic and extradesmosomic proteins demonstrate an overlap between dilated heart disease, arrhythmogenic cardiomyopathy, and channelopathies, with expressions of different phenotypes.

Mutations affecting compound area genes are now considered to be important in the pathogenesis of these diseases, which could represent a continuum between them from a purely arrhythmogenic phenotype to one with left ventricular dilation and congestive failure.

The canine patient in this report had conditions that suggested the presence of a canalopathy, given that the corrected QT interval was prolonged and had structural alterations suggestive of Arrhythmogenic Cardiomyopathy, such as fibroadipose replacement [22]. It also presented signs that are frequently seen in dilated cardiomyopathy such as undulating myocardial fibers. This indicates that further studies are required to differentiate between these different phenotypic presentations.

In the case presented in the feline, the changes were totally limited to the free wall of the left ventricle, but although the damage was transmural, a small layer of the subendocardial was preserved. Since transmural heart attack of epicardial coronary origin has not been described and no coronary pathology has been found in the arteries that supplied the fibrofatty replacement segment in the feline left ventricle, the hypothesis that it is an ischemic pathology would be discarded. It is also important to note that in the rest of the feline heart that was preserved without injury, there was no hypertrophy, which suggests that we can also rule out the terminal phase of feline hypertrophic cardiomyopathy, where there may be thinning of the wall due to microvascular injury. In the latter case, in the final stage of hypertrophic heart disease with abnormal remodeling, there is usually a lot of fibrosis. In our feline case, this is not true because there was a notorious fat replacement, which makes us think of an Arrhythmogenic Cardiomyopathy of the left ventricle.

8. Conclusion

In both of the presented cases, the lesions by fatty tissue replacement of the cardiac muscle in the left ventricular wall, without evidence of coronary ischemic lesion or of microvascular lesion, allow us to conclude that the compatible diagnosis is Arrhythmogenic Cardiomyopathy. The clinical course of the canine, which did not present heart failure but did present severe arrhythmias, also speaks in favor of Arrhythmogenic Cardiomyopathy. In the case of the feline patient, it was similar to the canine patient and the histopathological findings of fatty replacement in the ventricle were similar in both animals.

To the authors' knowledge, this report is the first one made about Left Ventricle Arrythmogenic Cardiomyopathy in companion animals, and future studies are required to better understand the disease in these species.

Author details

Guillermo Belerenian[1*], Cristian Daniel Rodríguez[2], Víctor Castillo[3] and Gustavo Abuin[4]

1 Instituto de Zoonosis Luis Pasteur (CABA), Companion Animals, Argentina

2 Companion Animals, Argentina

3 Instituto de Zoonosis Luis Pasteur (CABA), Argentina

4 Hospital de Agudos Fernandez (CABA), Argentina

*Address all correspondence to: cardiolibre2@gmail.com

References

[1] Corrado D, Link MS, Calkins H. Arrhythmogenic right ventricular cardiomyopathy. The New England Journal of Medicine. 2017;**376**(1):61-72

[2] Basso C, Fox PR, Meurs KM, Towbin JA, Spier AW, Calabrese F, et al. Arrhythmogenic right ventricular cardiomyopathy causing sudden cardiac death in boxer dogs: A new animal model of human disease. Circulation. 2004;**109**(9):1180-1185

[3] Belerenian G, Donati PA, Rodríguez CD, Castillo V, Guevara JM, Olivares RWI. Left-dominant arrhythmogenic cardiomyopathy in a Fila Brasileiro dog. Open Veterinary Journal. 2022;**12**(4):495-501. DOI: 10.5455/OVJ.2022.v12.i4.11

[4] Protonotarios A, Elliott PM. Arrhythmogenic cardiomyopathy: A disease or merely a phenotype? European Cardiology. 2020;**15**:1-5

[5] Calkins H, Tandri H. Left ventricular involvement in ARVD/C: Is it time to readjust our views? Circulation. Arrhythmia and Electrophysiology. 2015;**8**(6):1311-1312

[6] Berte B, Denis A, Amraoui S, Yamashita S, Komatsu Y, Pillois X, et al. Characterization of the left-sided substrate in Arrhythmogenic right ventricular cardiomyopathy. Circulation Arrhythmia and Electrophysiology. 2015;**8**(6):1403-1412

[7] Delmar M, McKenna WJ. The cardiac desmosome and arrhythmogenic cardiomyopathies: From gene to disease. Circulation Research. 2010;**107**(6):700-714

[8] Sheikh F, Ross RS, Chen J. Cell-cell connection to cardiac disease. Trends in Cardiovascular Medicine. 2009;**19**(6):182-190

[9] Sen-Chowdhry S, Syrris P, Prasad SK, Hughes SE, Merrifield R, Ward D, et al. Left-dominant arrhythmogenic cardiomyopathy: An under-recognized clinical entity. Journal of the American College of Cardiology. 2008;**52**(25):2175-2187

[10] Shen MT, Yang ZG, Diao KY, Jiang L, Zhang Y, Liu X, et al. Left ventricular involvement in arrhythmogenic right ventricular dysplasia/ cardiomyopathy predicts adverse clinical outcomes: A cardiovascular magnetic resonance feature tracking study. Scientific Reports. 2019;**9**(1):14235

[11] Lyon RC, Mezzano V, Wright AT, Pfeiffer E, Chuang J, Banares K, et al. Connexin defects underlie arrhythmogenic right ventricular cardiomyopathy in a novel mouse model. Human Molecular Genetics. 2014;**23**(5):1134-1150

[12] Mu J, Zhang G, Xue D, Xi M, Qi J, Dong H. Sudden cardiac death owing to arrhythmogenic right ventricular cardiomyopathy: Two case reports and systematic literature review. Medicine (Baltimore). 2017;**96**(47):e8808

[13] Hariu CD, Carpenter DH Jr. Arrhythmogenic right ventricular cardiomyopathy in boxers. Compendium: Continuing Education for Veterinarians. 2010;**32**(12):e3

[14] Harpster NK. Boxer cardiomyopathy. A review of the long-term benefits of antiarrhythmic therapy. The Veterinary Clinics of North America. Small Animal Practice. 1991;**21**(5):989-1004

[15] Palermo V, Stafford Johnson MJ, Sala E, Brambilla PG, Martin MWS. Cardiomyopathy in boxer dogs: A retrospective study of the clinical presentation, diagnostic findings and survival. Journal of Veterinary Cardiology. 2011;**13**(1):45-55

[16] Nakao S, Hirakawa A, Yamamoto S, Kobayashi M, Machida N. Pathological features of arrhythmogenic right ventricular cardiomyopathy in middle-aged dogs. The Journal of Veterinary Medical Science. 2011;**73**(8):1031-1036

[17] Orgeron GM, Crosson JE. Arrhythmogenic right ventricular dysplasia/cardiomyopathy. Cardiol. Young. 2017;**27**(S1):S57-S61

[18] Stadiotti I, Catto V, Casella M, Tondo C, Pompilio G, Sommariva E. Arrhythmogenic cardiomyopathy: The guilty party in adipogenesis. Journal of Cardiovascular Translational Research. 2017;**10**(5-6):446-454

[19] Xu T, Yang Z, Vatta M, Rampazzo A, Beffagna G, Pillichou K, et al. Compound and digenic heterozygosity contributes to arrhythmogenic right ventricular cardiomyopathy. Journal of the American College of Cardiology. 2010;**55**(6):587-597

[20] Yoo SJ, Grosse-Wortmann L, Hamilton RM. Magnetic resonance imaging assessment of arrhythmogenic right ventricular cardiomyopathy/dysplasia in children. Korean Circulation Journal. 2010;**40**(8):357-367

[21] Tavano A, Maurel B, Gaubert JY, Varoquaux A, Cassagneau P, Vidal V, et al. MR imaging of arrhythmogenic right ventricular dysplasia: What the radiologist needs to know. Diagnostic and Interventional Imaging. 2015;**96**(5):449-460

[22] Fernández-Falgueras A, Sarquella-Brugada G, Brugada J, Brugada R, Campuzano O. Cardiac channelopathies and sudden death: Recent clinical and genetic advances. Biology (Basel). 2017;**6**(1):7

Chapter 7

Premature Ventricular Complex-Induced/–Aggravated Cardiomyopathy

Mustafa Kaplangoray

Abstract

Premature Ventricular Complexes-induced Cardiomyopathy (PVC-CM) is a cardiomyopathy characterized by left ventricular (LV) dysfunction caused by frequent premature ventricular complexes (PVCs), with the potential for resolution with treatment. Although the mechanism of PVC-CM development involves various cellular and intercellular mechanisms along with multiple risk factors, its mechanism has not been fully elucidated. In patients who develop symptomatic and/or LV dysfunction, suppression of PVCs is indicated for treatment. Despite the use of antiarrhythmic drugs in treatment, hesitations regarding their use persist due to common side effects, including proarrhythmia. Recently introduced radiofrequency ablation therapy is both effective and has a high success rate when performed by experienced hands, and current guidelines recommend it as the first option for patients developing LV dysfunction. This review will discuss PVC-CM in detail, alongside current guidelines and studies.

Keywords: ablation, induced cardiomyopathy, left ventricular dysfunction, premature ventrucular complex, premature ventricular contraction-induced cardiomyopathy, heart failure

1. Introduction

Premature ventricular complexes (PVCs) were first described by the French physiologist Étienne-Jules Marey in the early 1800s. Marey was the first to obtain an electrocardiographic recording in animals using a capillary electrometer, through which he also described PVCs. The first electrocardiography (ECG) recording in humans was made shortly after Marey by Augustus Desiré Waller in 1887. Subsequent years saw significant advancements in the identification, significance, and treatment of arrhythmias, paralleled by technological developments and the introduction of Holter monitoring technology developed by American biophysicist Norman J. Holter [1]. PVCs are a common type of ventricular arrhythmia, and their prognostic significance is closely related to underlying cardiac diseases. For years, PVCs were considered benign in individuals without any structural heart disease. However, between the 1970s and 1980s, frequent PVCs observed post-myocardial infarction (MI) were claimed to trigger ventricular tachycardia (VT), ventricular fibrillation (VF), and sudden cardiac death, suggesting the necessity for PVC suppression therapy [2].

In the Cardiac Arrhythmia Suppression Trial (CAST), treatment of PVCs with antiarrhythmic drugs in patients who had previously experienced an MI, although successful in suppressing PVCs, was associated with increased mortality [3]. Despite the findings of this study, recent studies have shown that PVCs can cause cardiomyopathy and heart failure, and effective treatment of PVCs is associated with recovery in cardiac functions [4, 5]. PVC-induced cardiomyopathy (PVC-CM) is defined as LV dysfunction caused by frequent PVCs, with the potential for improvement with PVC suppression therapy. The absence of any underlying structural heart disease is important for differential diagnosis, making PVC-induced cardiomyopathy a sort of diagnosis of exclusion.

2. Epidemiology and prevalence

Before discussing the prevalence of PVC-CM, it would be better to examine the prevalence of PVCs, which are involved in the etiology of this cardiomyopathy. Data on the prevalence of PVCs come from ECG databases and Holter monitoring records intended for treatment purposes and have seen an increasing incidence in recent years. In a comprehensive community-based study involving 122,034 US Air Force personnel, where 48-second ECG records were collected, the frequency of PVCs was observed to be 7.8 per 1000 individuals and was found to increase with age [6]. In a more recent multi-ethnic cohort (ARIC [Atherosclerosis Risk in Communities] study), among 14,000 participants without a diagnosis of heart failure and based on a 10-second ECG record, the frequency of PVCs was found to be 1.8% [7]. The Cardiovascular Health Study, involving 4710 individuals aged over 65 and similarly based on a 10-second ECG record in a population-based cohort excluding heart failure patients, found the frequency of PVCs to be 5.2% [7]. It is not surprising that the prevalence of PVCs increases with longer monitoring durations. Indeed, in the ARIC study, while the prevalence was 5.5% in a 2-minute ECG record, the Framingham Heart Study found a 12% prevalence of PVCs and other complex ventricular arrhythmias in a 1-hour ECG monitoring of individuals without coronary artery disease [8, 9]. In a community-based cohort in Lichtenstein, among individuals aged 24–41 undergoing 24-hour Holter monitoring, at least one PVC was found in 69%, with a median of 2 PVCs, and the 95th percentile was 193 PVCs [10].

While a PVC burden of >24% has been proposed to have the highest sensitivity and specificity (79% and 78%, respectively) for predicting the development of PVC-CM, recent studies have suggested that this rate could be lower [5]. However, the latest guidelines on ventricular tachycardia by the ESC indicate that the minimum PVC burden for the development of PVC-CM is 10%, with the risk increasing above 20% [11].

Although there is no consensus on the prevalence of PVC-CM, it is estimated to be higher than reported, with a prevalence of approximately 7% in patients with a PVC burden of >10% [12]. Clinical studies have reported the frequency of PVC-CM in patients referred for radiofrequency ablation (RFA) due to PVCs to be between 9% and 30% [5, 13, 14]. The CHF-STAT (Survival Trial of Antiarrhythmic Therapy in Congestive Heart Failure) study demonstrated that PVC-CM (LVEF <40% and > 10 PVCs/h) accounted for 40% of all cardiomyopathy patients [15].

3. Mechanism and pathophysiology

Compared to tachycardia-induced cardiomyopathy, the cellular-level mechanism of PVC-CM is unclear. However, it is evident that the histopathological and cellular characteristics of PVC-CM differ from other forms of heart failure [16]. A more comprehensive evaluation from both a cellular level and clinical perspective is necessary to fully understand the mechanism.

The proposed mechanisms related to PVC-CM at the cellular level are speculative and based on animal models. Studies conducted by Wang et al. [17] in a dog model have shown that prolongation of the action potential duration and beat-to-beat variability in the action potential lead to a decrease in inward and outward (L-type calcium) currents, causing repolarization heterogeneity. These results could potentially increase the risk of sudden cardiac death by leading to triggered activity and malignant arrhythmias. Additionally, the study highlighted that the contractile dysfunction observed in PVC-CM could be explained by alterations in calcium-induced calcium release in the sarcoplasm. Another study in a dog model showed that the impairment in LVEF caused by PVCs only became apparent after three months, supporting the notion that the mechanism in PVC-CM might be more functional than structural, as myocardial fibrosis and apoptosis are observed to be minimal or absent [18, 19].

From a clinical perspective, the theory of mechanical ventricular dyssynchrony secondary to abnormal electrical activity may be a more solid theory [20, 21]. The impairment in LV function caused by left bundle branch block and right ventricular pacing is a similar example. In both cases, changes in myocardial blood flow are observed alongside asymmetrically increased wall thickness in areas activated late [22, 23].

4. Predictive factors for PVC-CM

Not all patients with PVCs develop PVC-CM, and some patients with a high burden of PVCs continue their lives symptom-free and without any impairment in LV function. Given this situation, certain predisposing factors that could play a role in the development of PVC-CM have naturally come to the forefront. We will now discuss these factors.

4.1 Characteristics of premature ventricular complexes

The QRS duration of PVCs ≥140 ms has been reported in many studies as an independent factor for the impairment of LV functions (**Figure 1**). These PVCs predominantly originate from the free wall or outflow tract [24–27]. In contrast, PVCs originating from the fascicles and septum tend to have a narrower QRS duration. Additionally, a small-scale study has identified interpolated PVCs and PVC burden as predisposing factors for the development of PVC-CM [28].

PVCs with a short coupling interval have been associated with idiopathic ventricular fibrillation [29]. Several studies have shown that interpolated PVCs and short coupling intervals, especially below 450 ms, are associated with low LVEF and pose a risk for the development of PVC-CM. Furthermore, the dispersion of the PVC coupling interval is also known to be a significant factor in the development of PVC-CM (**Figure 2**) [28, 30].

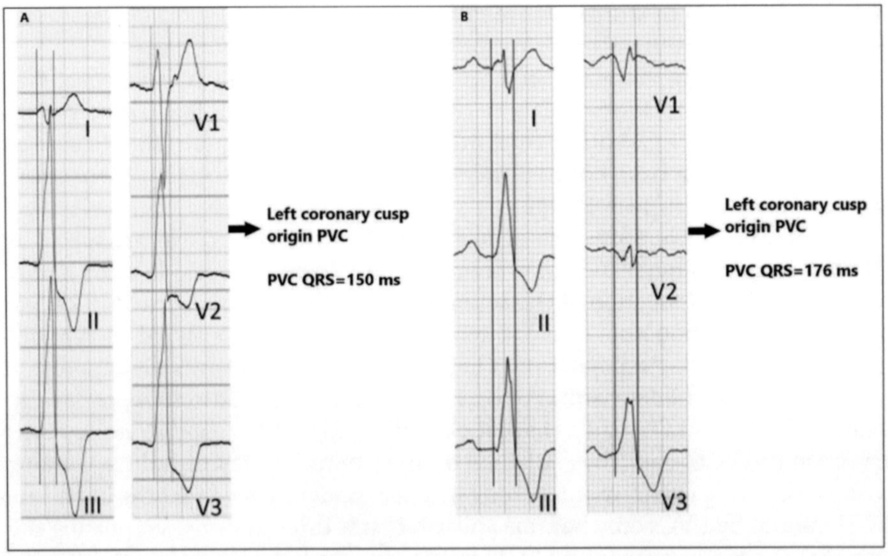

Figure 1.
VPC QRS durations of patients with similar origin and PVC burden. A: PVC-QRS duration is 150 ms and left ventricular functions are normal. B: PVC-QRS duration is 176 ms and left ventricular ejection fraction is 40% and ECG example of the case that progressed to PVC-CM [16].

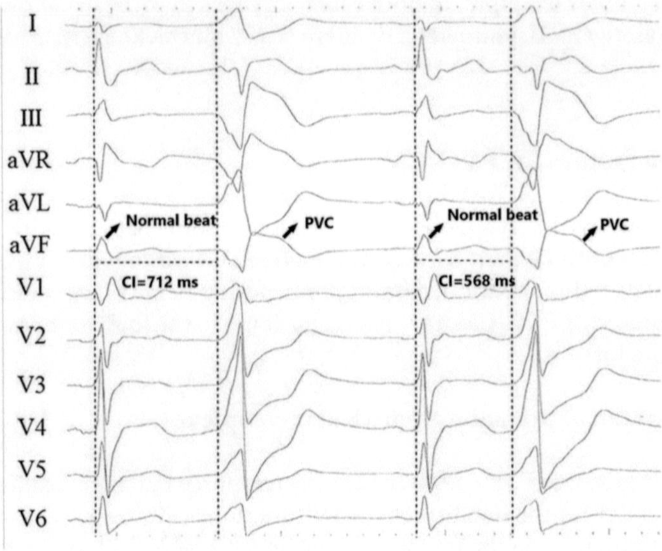

Figure 2.
In the ECG sample of the patient with PVC-CM, CI dispersion was measured as 144 ms (threshold value for PVC-CM development is >99 ms) [16].

4.2 Premature ventricular complex burden

The burden of PVCs is considered a major factor in the development of PVC-CM. In two major studies, a PVC burden of >16% and > 24% has been accepted as the threshold for the development of PVC-CM (with sensitivity and specificity of 79–100% and 78–87%, respectively). However, other studies have considered a minimum threshold of 10% for the development of PVC-CM, as improvements in LV function have been observed in patients with a PVC burden between 6–8%. In this context, the duration of ambulatory ECG monitoring is critically important, and when the monitoring period is maintained between 24 hours to 7 days, the number of patients reaching the 10% threshold doubles [16].

4.3 Origin of premature ventricular complexes

Del Carpio et al. demonstrated that PVCs originating from the right ventricle (RV) caused impairment in LV function with a lower daily burden of PVCs compared to those originating from the LV [25]. This could be due to greater LV dyssynchrony in RV-originating PVCs. Additionally, recent studies have shown that PVCs of epicardial origin have a higher risk of developing cardiomyopathy. As previously mentioned, this may be attributed to greater mechanical dyssynchrony in epicardial-originating PVCs [21]. Given this, detailed ECG evaluations to predict PVC localization before potential radiofrequency ablation (RFA) treatment are of great importance. Below is a brief algorithm that may be useful for PVC localization.

PVCs originating from the ventricular outflow tract musculature, especially from the RV outflow tract, are responsible for two-thirds of all idiopathic PVCs [25]. These originate from points where the myocardial tissue extends towards the aortic and pulmonary valves. The remaining one-third originate from various points such as the septum, papillary muscle, free wall, and ventricular fascicles. Outflow tract-originating PVCs have an inferior axis on surface ECG, visible with positive QRS morphology in leads II, III, and aVF. Those originating from the RV outflow tract generally exhibit a left bundle branch block pattern, though it should not be forgotten that those originating from the aortic cusp can also display the same morphology. On the other hand, the presence of a right bundle branch block morphology supports the origin of PVCs from the LV. However, it is crucial to remember that the outflow tract anatomy of the heart is complex and should be considered in three dimensions. In this context, ECG-based evaluations also gain importance in addition to these criteria.

- A later transition of the QRS in precordial leads compared to the transition in normal sinus rhythm should suggest PVCs originating from the right ventricular outflow tract, and the converse may also be true. The more anterior the origin, the later the transition zone in the precordials will be [31, 32]. If both the sinus rhythm and PVCs show QRS transition in V3, then the R transition ratio can be indicative; if the ratio of the R wave in PVCs in V2 to the R wave in sinus rhythm is $\geq$0.6, then the PVCs are located on the left side with 95% sensitivity and 100% specificity [33].

- Another criterion used to determine the location of PVCs is the maximum deflection index, which is the ratio of the maximum QRS deflection duration to the total QRS duration. If this index is above 0.55, the PVCs are likely to be of epicardial origin (**Figure 3**) [25].

4.4 Variability circadian PVCs

Circadian variability of PVCs is considered an independent risk factor for the development of PVC-CM [35]. A recent study showed that PVCs exhibiting circadian variation have a high likelihood of being induced in the electrophysiology laboratory.

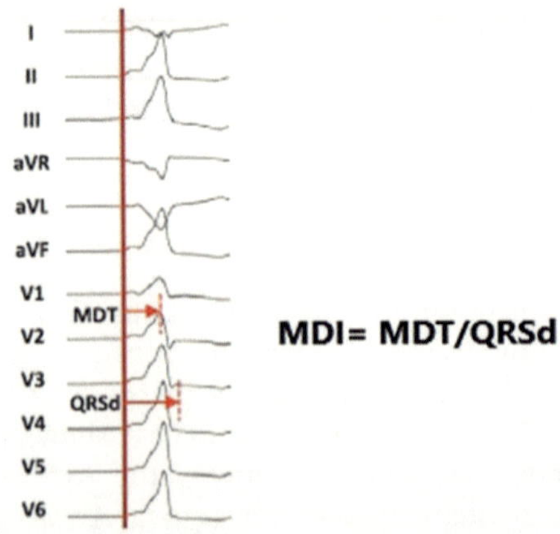

Figure 3.
Calculation of maximum deflection index (MDI). It is obtained by dividing the QRS deflection duration by the QRS duration. In this case, MDI was measured as 0.64 [34].

Additionally, individuals with a high heart rate due to PVCs responded to isoproterenol during electrophysiological studies, and these patients also had a high success rate for RFA [36]. However, the success of the procedure is lower in patients in whom there is no correlation between PVCs burden and average heart rate.

4.5 Gender

Latchamsetty et al. demonstrated that male gender is an independent risk factor for the development of PVC-CM [14]. Surksha et al. found that while the incidence of symptomatic PVCs is higher in women, the incidence of PVC-CM is similar between genders [37]. It should not be forgotten that symptoms leading to early diagnosis and thereby early initiation of treatment in symptomatic individuals may prevent the development of cardiomyopathy. The perception of symptoms in women could be a factor leading to earlier treatment initiation. The role of gender in the development of PVC-CM could also be due to hormonal differences, making this an area worthy of further research today [38].

4.6 Genetics

The fact that PVC-CM develops in some patients with a similar PVC burden while others remain unaffected suggests a genetic predisposition. For example, the faulty variation R222Q of the Nav1.5 subunit of the sodium channel, causing large and early sodium current, is thought to contribute to the rate of Purkinje-originating PVCs. This same mutation has also been shown to play a role in the response of patients with PVC-CM cardiomyopathy to amiodarone or flecainide [39].

5. Clinical presentation and diagnostic approach

The duration for the development of PVC-CM is unclear; it may span days or months [40–42]. In animal experiments, the development of PVC-CM has been observed within 4 weeks under continuous and high PVC burden (daily PVC burden >30%) [19, 43]. The uncertainty of the onset time and variation in PVC burden in humans make it difficult to estimate this duration.

Patients with PVC-CM may present asymptomatic or with symptoms of heart failure. Palpitations are the most common symptom among these patients. The PVC coupling interval is considered a significant factor in symptomatology, and patients with a PVC coupling interval < 0.5 are mostly symptomatic [44]. A detailed history and thorough physical examination are important factors in differential diagnosis. Apart from regular pulse, variable intensity of heart sounds, and mild signs of heart failure, specific findings may not be observed during the physical examination. The diagnosis of PVC-CM can be considered a diagnosis of exclusion, especially in patients with nonischemic cardiomyopathy and a PVC burden >10%. Another critical point is distinguishing whether PVCs are an etiology or secondary to an underlying cardiomyopathy. If PVCs are the consequence of cardiomyopathy and are frequent, they can worsen heart failure and symptoms, referred to as "PVCs-aggravated cardiomyopathy" [45, 46]. Echocardiography and PVC morphology play a significant role in differential diagnosis (**Table 1**).

ECG and prolonged ambulatory ECG monitoring are fundamental tools for diagnosis. Loring et al. suggest that a minimum of 6 days of monitoring is necessary to maximize the detection of PVC burden [47]. Correspondingly, nearly half of potential PVC-CM patients may be missed in the conventional 24-hour ambulatory ECG monitoring [47].

PVC-CM does not have specific echocardiographic findings, but mild to moderate LV ejection fraction (LVEF) impairment, LV dilatation, mild mitral regurgitation, and left atrial dilatation are commonly observed echocardiographic findings. Improvements in these findings are generally seen weeks after PVC suppression therapy [16]. Cardiac imaging is an important diagnostic tool in patients with a PVC burden >10% and should be performed promptly. Cardiac magnetic resonance (CMR) imaging can identify scar or fibrosis load through late-gadolinium enhancement (LGE). Scar load is considered a significant parameter in response to PVC suppression therapy [48]. In subclinical PVC-CMP forms (LVEF ≥50%), speckle tracking has shown improvement in radial,

	PVC-aggravated cardiomyopathies	**PVC-CM**
Patient characteristics	Older and have known heart disease	Healthy otherwise
Comorbidities	CAD, other types of cardiomyopathy, hypertension	No cardiac disease
Echocardiogram	Segmental hypokinesis, LVEF <25%	Global hypokinesis, LVEF 37 ± 10%
Cardiac magnetic resonance imaging (late-gadolinium enhancement)	Significant scar	Absence or minimal scar burden
PVC frequency	<5000/24 h (<5%)	≥ 10,000/24 h (≥ 10%)
PVC pattern	Multifocal	Monomorphic
QRS morphology	Nonspecific	RVOT/LVOT/epicardial
Response to PVC suppression	No change in LV function	Improvement of LV function

CAD: coronary artery disease; RVOT: right ventricular outflow tract; LVOT: left ventricular outflow tract.

Table 1.
Clinical, electrocardiographic and imaging features of PVC-CM and PVC-aggravated cardiomyopathies.

Recommendation	Class	Level
Diagnostic evaluation		
In patients with an unexplained reduced EF and a PVC burden of at least 10%, PVC-induced cardiomyopathy should be considered	IIa	C
In patients with suspected PVC-induced cardiomyopathy, CMR should be considered	IIa	B
Treatment		
In patients with a cardiomyopathy suspected to be caused by frequent and predominately monomorphic PVCs, catheter ablation is recommended	I	C
In patients with a cardiomyopathy suspected to be caused by frequent and predominately monomorphic PVCs, treatment with AADs[a] should be considered if catheter ablation is not desired, suspected to be high-risk, or unsuccessful	IIa	C
In patients with SHD in whom predominately monomorphic frequent PVCs are suspected to be contributing to the cardiomyopathy, AAD (amiodarone) treatment or catheter ablation should be considered.	IIa	B
In non-responders to CRT with frequent, predominately monomorphic PVCs limiting optimal biventricular pacing despite pharmacological therapy, catheter ablation or AADs should be considered.	IIa	C

AAD, anti-arrhythmic drug; CMR, cardiac magnetic resonance; CRT, cardiac resynchronization therapy; EF, ejection fraction; ICD, implantable cardioverter defibrillator; LV, left ventricular; PVC, premature ventricular complex; SHD, structural heart disease.[a]Flecainide only in selected patients (ICD recipients, only moderate LV dysfunction)

Table 2.
In the 2022 ESC guidelines for the management of patients with ventricular arrhythmias and the prevention of sudden cardiac death, there are diagnostic evaluation and treatment recommendations for cardiomyopathies induced or exacerbated by premature ventricular complexes.

circumferential, and longitudinal strains after RFA therapy [49, 50]. These findings are consistent with translational studies showing a mild and linear decrease in LV systolic functions at PVC burdens of 7%, 14%, and 25% [43].

In recent years, myocarditis has been proposed to trigger frequent PVCs and cardiomyopathy. Increased hs-CRP has been reported as an independent factor for PVCs in the Chinese population [51, 52]. Therefore, whether inflammatory processes are a cause or consequence of PVCs remains unclear.

As mentioned earlier, PVCs can cause impairment in LV functions in those with structural heart disease. It should not be forgotten that in patients with structural heart disease undergoing CRT implantation, PVCs can reduce the effectiveness of optimal CRT. In differential diagnosis, a small left ventricular diastolic diameter and a short QRS complex duration support the diagnosis of PVC-CM. CMR is a valuable diagnostic tool in differentiating PVC-CM from PVC-aggravated cardiomyopathy, with the presence of LGE supporting the latter diagnosis. Additionally, PVCs with a right bundle branch block pattern show a strong correlation with LGE, and CMR is recommended in these patients. Another way to distinguish PVC-CM from PVC-aggravated cardiomyopathy is that PVC-CM shows improvement after PVC suppression therapy (**Tables 1** and 2) [11].

6. Treatment

Currently, treating patients with PVC-CM with RFA or antiarrhythmic drug therapy (AAD) is a widely accepted strategy [53]. However, the situation is not as clear in asymptomatic individuals with a PVC burden >10% without life-threatening arrhythmias. Data on this group of patients is limited, and even if asymptomatic, they should be closely monitored every 6 to 12 months. If any heart failure symptoms develop, prolonged ambulatory ECG monitoring and echocardiography should be performed. Although there is no assessment of spontaneously resolving PVCs, the CHF-STAT study showed significant improvements in PVC burden in 12% of patients in the placebo group after 6 months [15].

An 80% reduction in PVC burden from the initial load indicates the real effect of the treatment [54], as spontaneous changes in PVC burden are not expected at this rate. It should be noted that these criteria are based on 24-hour ambulatory ECG monitoring data, and data from longer-term monitoring are limited. As mentioned at the beginning, RFA and AAD therapy are recommended for PVC suppression treatment today, and both treatment options have nearly the same success rate (70–80%) [16].

The success rate of RFA is lower for PVCs originating from the papillary muscle, epicardium, near the coronary artery, and the conduction system [14, 30, 55]. Therefore, 5–15% of patients may need AAD therapy after RFA [14]. PVC suppression therapy, both AAD and RFA, carries a low risk. The complication rate with RFA is between 5–8%, while the discontinuation rate of AADs due to long-term side effects is around 10% [56].

Randomized clinical trials of AADs in this field date back to a time before PVC-CM was defined. The Cardiac Arrhythmia Suppression Trial (CAST) demonstrated that class IC AADs used in patients with frequent PVCs following acute myocardial infarction increased mortality. However, studies such as the GESICA (Grupo de Estudio de la Sobrevida en la Insuficiencia Cardiaca en Argentina), CAMIAT (Canadian Amiodarone Myocardial Infarction Arrhythmia Trial), and CHF-STAT have indicated that amiodarone treatment post-acute myocardial infarction and in nonischemic cardiomyopathies showed a trend towards reduced mortality [15, 57].

Currently, there are no randomized studies comparing RFA and AAD treatments. However, a recent retrospective study showed a greater reduction in PVC burden with RFA treatment compared to AAD treatment (mean reduction: RFA 15.5 ± 1.3% vs. AADs 4.8 ± 0.8; $p < 0.001$). A single-center small study also demonstrated that RFA treatment was more effective in patients with a low PVC burden [30].

After PVC suppression therapy, improvements in left ventricular function, left ventricular dilatation, and mitral regurgitation have been observed, along with a decrease in BNP levels. Even in superimposed cardiomyopathies, RFA treatment has resulted in an increase in LVEF of between 10–15% [16]. A recent multicenter study of 245 patients with nonischemic cardiomyopathy and frequent PVCs showed that RFA treatment improved left ventricular functions in 67% of the patients [58].

The success rate of RFA for PVC suppression therapy today ranges between 90–75%. Therefore, the latest ESC arrhythmia guidelines recommend RFA as the first option for treating PVC-CM. The success rate of RFA is related to the origin of PVCs (highest for outflow tract PVCs), diversity of PVC morphology, and the presence of late gadolinium enhancement (LGE) on CMR [11].

AADs used in PVC suppression therapy have also been shown to increase LVEF. A randomized study demonstrated that amiodarone provided more PVC suppression and was associated with greater improvements in LVEF compared to placebo [59]. Sodium channel blockers are also effective agents in PVC suppression therapy [30]. One study showed that treatment with flecainide reduced the PVC burden from 36–10% and increased LVEF from 37–49% [56]. However, it should not be forgotten that flecainide's organ toxicities and its use post-acute myocardial infarction have been associated with increased mortality [34]. In selected patients with PVC-CM or PVC-aggravated CMP and those implanted with ICDs, flecainide may be considered an option for PVC suppression therapy.

7. Conclusion

PVC-CM is a type of cardiomyopathy with a unique pathophysiology that can be fully corrected with treatment. A detailed patient history, 12-lead ECG, Holter-ECG (preferably long-term), echocardiography, and CMR are fundamental tools for the diagnosis of this cardiomyopathy. The development of PVC-CM requires a minimum PVC burden of at least 10%, and the risk increases further when the PVC burden exceeds 20%. Although there is an option for AAD or RFA treatment for PVCs, RFA, which is more effective especially in cases with developed LV dysfunction, should be considered the primary option.

Author details

Mustafa Kaplangoray
Medical Faculty, Department of Cardiology, Şeyh Edebali University, Bilecik, Turkey

*Address all correspondence to: mkaplangoray@gmail.com

References

[1] Latchamsetty R, Bogun F. Premature ventricular complexes and premature ventricular complex induced cardiomyopathy. Current Problems in Cardiology. 2015;**40**(9):379-422

[2] Panizo JG, Barra S, Mellor G, Heck P, Agarwal S. Premature ventricular complex-induced cardiomyopathy. Arrhythmia and electrophysiology Review. 2018;**7**(2):128

[3] Echt DS, Liebson PR, Mitchell LB, et al. Mortality and morbidity in patients receiving encainide, flecainide, or placebo The Cardiac Arrhythmia Suppression Trial. The New England Journal of Medicine. 1991;**324**:781-788. DOI: 10.1056/ NEJM199103213241201

[4] Yarlagadda RK, Iwai S, Stein KM, et al. Reversal of cardiomyopathy in patients with repetitive monomorphic ventricular ectopy originating from the right ventricular outflow tract. Circulation. 2005;**112**:1092-1097. DOI: 10.1161/ CIRCULATIONAHA.105.546432

[5] Baman TS, Lange DC, Ilg KJ, et al. Relationship between burden of premature ventricular complexes and left ventricular function. Heart Rhythm. 2010;7:865-869. DOI: 10.1016/j. hrthm.2010.03.036

[6] Hiss RG, Lamb LE. Electrocardiographic findings in 122,043 individuals. Circulation. 1962;**25**:947-961. DOI: 10.1161/01.cir.25.6.947

[7] Nguyen KT, Vittinghoff E, Dewland TA, Dukes JW, Soliman EZ, Stein PK, et al. Ectopy on a single 12-lead ECG, incident cardiac myopathy, and death in the community. Journal of the American Heart Association. 2017;**6**:e006028

[8] Agarwal SK, Simpson RJ Jr, Rautaharju P, Alonso A, Shahar E, Massing M, et al. Relation of ventricular premature complexes to heart failure (from the atherosclerosis risk In communities [ARIC] study). The American Journal of Cardiology. 2012;**109**:105-109. DOI: 10.1016/j. amjcard.2011.08.009

[9] Bikkina M, Larson MG, Levy D. Prognostic implications of asymptomatic ventricular arrhythmias: The Framingham heart study. Annals of Internal Medicine. 1992;**117**:990-996. DOI: 10.7326/0003-4819-117-12-990

[10] von Rotz M, Aeschbacher S, Bossard M, Schoen T, Blum S, Schneider S, et al. Risk factors for premature ventricular contractions in young and healthy adults. Heart. 2017;**103**:702-707. DOI: 10.1136/ heartjnl-2016-309632

[11] Zeppenfeld K, Tfelt-Hansen J, De Riva M, Winkel BG, Behr ER, Blom NA, et al. 2022 ESC guidelines for the management of patients with ventricular arrhythmias and the prevention of sudden cardiac death: Developed by the task force for the management of patients with ventricular arrhythmias and the prevention of sudden cardiac death of the European Society of Cardiology (ESC) endorsed by the Association for European Paediatric and Congenital Cardiology (AEPC). European Heart Journal. 2022;**43**(40):3997-4126

[12] Hasdemir C, Ulucan C, Yavuzgil O, et al. Tachycardia-induced cardiomyopathy in patients with idiopathic ventricular arrhythmias: The incidence, clinical and electrophysiologic characteristics, and

the predictors. Journal of Cardiovascular Electrophysiology. 2011;**22**:663-668

[13] Hasdemir C, Yuksel A, Camli D, et al. Late gadolinium enhancement CMR in patients with tachycardia-induced cardiomyopathy caused by idiopathic ventricular arrhythmias. Pacing and Clinical Electrophysiology. 2012;**35**:465-470

[14] Latchamsetty R, Yokokawa M, Morady F, et al. Multicenter outcomes for catheter ablation of idiopathic premature ventricular complexes. Journal of the American College of Cardiology. 2015;**1**:116-123

[15] Huizar JF, Fisher SG, Kaszala K, et al. Amiodarone is an effective treatment of PVCcardiomyopathy in the veteran population (abstr). Circulation. 2017;**136**(Suppl. 1):14667

[16] Huizar JF, Ellenbogen KA, Tan AY, Kaszala K. Arrhythmia-induced cardiomyopathy: JACC state-of-the-art review. Journal of the American College of Cardiology. 2019;**73**(18):2328-2344

[17] Wang Y, Eltit JM, Kaszala K, et al. Cellular mechanism of premature ventricular contraction–induced cardiomyopathy. Heart Rhythm. 2014;**11**:2064-2072. DOI: 10.1016/j.hrthm.2014.07.022

[18] Akoum NW, Daccarett M, Wasmund SL, Hamdan MH. An animal model for ectopy-induced cardiomyopathy. Pacing and Clinical Electrophysiology. 2011;**34**:291-295. DOI: 10.1111/j.1540-8159.2010.02947.x

[19] Huizar JF, Kaszala K, Potfay J, et al. Left ventricular systolic dysfunction induced by ventricular ectopy: A novel model for premature ventricular contraction-induced cardiomyopathy. Circulation. Arrhythmia and Electrophysiology. 2011;**4**:543-549. DOI: 10.1161/CIRCEP.111.962381

[20] Bogun F, Crawford T, Reich S, et al. Radiofrequency ablation of frequent, idiopathic premature ventricular complexes: Comparison with a control group without intervention. Heart Rhythm. 2007;**4**:863-867. DOI: 10.1016/j.hrthm.2007.03.003

[21] Latchamsetty R, Bogun F. Premature ventricular complexinduced cardiomyopathy. Revista Espanola de Cardiologia (Engl Ed). 2016;**69**:365-369. DOI: 10.1016/j.rec.2015.12.015

[22] Blanc JJ, Fatemi M, Bertault V, et al. Evaluation of left bundle branch block as a reversible cause of non-ischaemic dilated cardiomyopathy with severe heart failure. A new concept of left ventricular dyssynchrony-induced cardiomyopathy. Europace. 2005;7:604-610. DOI: 10.1016/j.eupc.2005.06.005

[23] Gardiwal A, Yu H, Oswald H, et al. Right ventricular pacing is an independent predictor for ventricular tachycardia/ventricular fibrillation occurrence and heart failure events in patients with an implantable cardioverter–defibrillator. Europace. 2008;**10**:358-363. DOI: 10.1093/europace/eun019

[24] Tantengco MV, Thomas RL, Karpawich PP. Left ventricular dysfunction after long-term right ventricular apical pacing in the young. Journal of the American College of Cardiology. 2001;**37**:2093-2100. DOI: 10.1016/S0735-1097(01)01302-X

[25] Del Carpio MF, Syed FF, Noheria A, et al. Characteristics of premature ventricular complexes as correlates of reduced left ventricular systolic function: Study of the burden, duration, coupling interval,

morphology and site of origin of PVCs. Journal of Cardiovascular Electrophysiology. 2011;**22**:791-798. DOI: 10.1111/j.1540-8167.2011.02021.x

[26] Yokokawa M, Kim HM, Good E, et al. Impact of QRS duration of frequent premature ventricular complexes on the development of cardiomyopathy. Heart Rhythm. 2012;**9**:1460-1464. DOI: 10.1016/j.hrthm.2012.04.036

[27] Moulton KP, Medcalf T, Lazzara R. Premature ventricular complex morphology. A marker for left ventricular structure and function. Circulation. 1990;**81**:1245-1251. DOI: 10.1161/01.CIR.81.4.1245

[28] Olgun H, Yokokawa M, Baman T, et al. The role of interpolation in PVC-induced cardiomyopathy. Heart Rhythm. 2011;**8**:1046-1049. DOI: 0.1016/j.hrthm.2011.02.034

[29] Knecht S, Sacher F, Wright M, et al. Long-term follow-up of idiopathic ventricular fibrillation ablation: A multicenter study. Journal of the American College of Cardiology. 2009;**54**:522-528

[30] Zhong L, Lee YH, Huang XM, et al. Relative efficacy of catheter ablation vs antiarrhythmic drugs in treating premature ventricular contractions: A single-center retrospective study. Heart Rhythm. 2014;**11**:187-193

[31] Scanavacca M, Lara S, Hardy C, Pisani CF. How to identify and treat epicardial origin of outflow tract tachycardias. Journal of Atrial Fibrillation. 2015;7:1195. DOI: 10.4022/jafib.1195

[32] Hutchinson MD, Garcia FC. An organized approach to the localization, mapping and ablation of outflow tract ventricular arrhythmias. Journal of Cardiovascular Electrophysiology. 2013;**24**:1189-1197. DOI: 10.1111/jce.12237

[33] Betensky BP, Park RE, Marchlinski FE, et al. The V(2) transition ratio: A new electrocardiographic criterion for distinguishing left from right ventricular outflow tract tachycardia origin. Journal of the American College of Cardiology. 2011;**57**:2255-2262. DOI: 10.1016/j.jacc.2011.01.035

[34] de Riva M, Watanabe M, Zeppenfeld K. Twelve-lead ECG of ventricular tachycardia in structural heart disease. Circulation: Arrhythmia and Electrophysiology. 2015;*8*(4):951-962

[35] Bas HD, Baser K, Hoyt J, et al. Effect of circadian variability in frequency of premature ventricular complexes on left ventricular function. Heart Rhythm. 2016;**13**:98-102. DOI: 10.1016/j.hrthm.2015.07.038

[36] Hamon D, Abehsira G, Gu K, et al. Circadian variability patterns predict and guide premature ventricular contraction ablation procedural inducibility and outcomes. Heart Rhythm. 2018;**15**:99-106. DOI: 10.1016/j.hrthm.2017.07.034

[37] Humphries KH, Kerr CR, Connolly SJ, et al. New-onset atrial fibrillation: Sex differences in presentation, treatment, and outcome. Circulation. 2001;**103**:2365-2370. DOI: 10.1161/01.CIR.103.19.2365

[38] Gwag HB, Kim EK, Hwang JK, et al. Is the stroke volume during post-ectopic beat associated with ventricular premature complex-related symptoms? Europace. 2017. DOI: 10.1093/europace/eux170

[39] Mann SA, Castro ML, Ohanian M, et al. R222Q SCN5A mutation is

associated with reversible ventricular ectopy and dilated cardiomyopathy. Journal of the American College of Cardiology. 2012;**60**:1566-1573

[40] Hamon D, Blaye-Felice MS, Bradfield JS, et al. A new combined parameter to predict premature ventricular complexes induced cardiomyopathy: Impact and recognition of epicardial origin. Journal of Cardiovascular Electrophysiology. 2016;**27**:709-717

[41] Ban JE, Park HC, Park JS, et al. Electrocardiographic and electrophysiological characteristics of premature ventricular complexes associated with left ventricular dysfunction in patients without structural heart disease. Europace. 2013;**15**:735-741

[42] Carballeira Pol L, Deyell MW, Frankel DS, et al. Ventricular premature depolarization QRS duration as a new marker of risk for the development of ventricular premature depolarization-induced cardiomyopathy. Heart Rhythm. 2014;**11**:299-306

[43] Tan AY, Hu YL, Potfay J, et al. Impact of ventricular ectopic burden in a premature ventricular contraction-induced cardiomyopathy animal model. Heart Rhythm. 2016;**13**:755-761

[44] Hwang JK, Park SJ, On YK, Kim JS, Park KM. Clinical characteristics and features of frequent idiopathic ventricular premature complexes in the Korean population. Korean Circulation Journal. 2015;**45**:391-397

[45] Sarrazin JF, Labounty T, Kuhne M, et al. Impact of radiofrequency ablation of frequent postinfarction premature ventricular complexes on left ventricular ejection fraction. Heart Rhythm. 2009;**6**:1543-1549

[46] El Kadri M, Yokokawa M, Labounty T, et al. Effect of ablation of frequent premature ventricular complexes on left ventricular function in patients with nonischemic cardiomyopathy. Heart Rhythm. 2015;**12**:706-713

[47] Loring Z, Hanna P, Pellegrini CN. Longer ambulatory ECG monitoring increases identification of clinically significant ectopy. Pacing and Clinical Electrophysiology. 2016;**39**:592-597

[48] Penela D, Martinez M, Fernandez-Armenta J, et al. Influence of myocardial scar on the response to frequent premature ventricular complex ablation. Heart. 2018

[49] Wijnmaalen AP, Delgado V, Schalij MJ, et al. Beneficial effects of catheter ablation on left ventricular and right ventricular function in patients with frequent premature ventricular contractions and preserved ejection fraction. Heart. 2010;**96**:1275-1280

[50] Yao J, Xu J, Yong YH, Cao KJ, Chen SL, Xu D. Evaluation of global and regional left ventricular systolic function in patients with frequent isolated premature ventricular complexes from the right ventricular outflow tract. Chinese Medical Journal. 2012;**125**:214-220

[51] Tung R, Bauer B, Schelbert H, et al. Incidence of abnormal positron emission tomography in patients with unexplained cardiomyopathy and ventricular arrhythmias: The potential role of occult inflammation in arrhythmogenesis. Heart Rhythm. 2015;**12**:2488-2498

[52] Chen Y, Wu S, Li W, et al. Higher highsensitivity c reactive protein is associated with future premature ventricular contraction: A community

based prospective cohort study. Scientific Reports. 2018;**8**:1-7

[53] Bozkurt B, Colvin M, Cook J, et al. Current diagnostic and treatment strategies for specific dilated cardiomyopathies: A scientific statement from the American Heart Association. Circulation. 2016;**134**:e579-e646

[54] Anastasiou-Nana MI, Menlove RL, Nanas JN, Anderson JL. Changes in spontaneous variability of ventricular ectopic activity as a function of time in patients with chronic arrhythmias. Circulation. 1988;**78**:286-295

[55] Maeda S, Chik WW, Liang JJ, et al. Recovery of renal dysfunction after catheter ablation of outflow tract ventricular arrhythmias in patients with ventricular premature depolarizationmediated cardiomyopathy. Journal of Interventional Cardiac Electrophysiology. 2017;**48**:43-50

[56] Hyman MC, Mustin D, Supple G, et al. Class IC antiarrhythmic drugs for suspected premature ventricular contraction-induced cardiomyopathy. Heart Rhythm. 2018;**15**:159-163

[57] Singh SN, Fletcher RD, Fisher SG, et al. Amiodarone in patients with congestive heart failure and asymptomatic ventricular arrhythmia. Survival trial of antiarrhythmic therapy in congestive heart failure. The New England Journal of Medicine. 1995;**333**:77-82

[58] Penela D, Acosta J, Aguinaga L, et al. Ablation of frequent PVC in patients meeting criteria for primary prevention ICD implant: Safety of withholding the implant. Heart Rhythm. 2015;**12**:2434-2442

[59] Echt DS, Liebson PR, Mitchell LB, Peters RW, Obias-Manno D, Barker AH, et al. Mortality and morbidity in patients receiving encainide, flecainide, or placebo. The cardiac arrhythmia suppression trial. The New England Journal of Medicine. 1991;**324**:781-788

Chapter 8

Comprehensive Interventions in End-Stage Cardiomyopathy: Mechanical Circulatory Support and Heart Transplantation

Alexandru Mihai Cornea, Guillermo Rodriguez and Alina Ligia Cornea

Abstract

This chapter provides a comprehensive exploration of the primary indications for employing mechanical circulatory support and heart transplantation in the treatment of end-stage cardiomyopathy. It emphasizes the specific types of support, patient selection criteria, optimal timing for intervention, and the prevalent varieties of mechanical assistance devices currently utilized. The chapter delves into nuanced patient outcomes concerning both temporary and long-term support, while also offering a succinct overview of the evolving perspectives within this field. Heart transplantation serves as the ultimate resource for cardiomyopathy patients for whom conventional medical therapy has proven ineffective. This section centers on delineating the indications and contraindications for heart transplantation, emphasizing patient care protocols, early and late postoperative complications, and the future trajectories in this domain. A critical analysis scrutinizes and compares the efficacy and applicability of mechanical assistance against heart transplantation within this patient cohort. Given the intricacies of surgical interventions for cardiomyopathy, the chapter outlines prospects, encompassing advancements such as xenotransplantation and the integration of new mechanical assist devices into the evolving landscape of treatments.

Keywords: cardiomyopathy, mechanical assist device, temporary circulatory support, donors after circulatory death, heart transplantation, xenotransplantation

1. Introduction

Cardiomyopathies (CMP) were initially characterized as myocardial diseases of unknown origin. Subsequently, the American Heart Association (AHA) redefined them as a diverse group of myocardial diseases linked to mechanical and or electrical dysfunction, which often manifest inappropriate ventricular hypertrophy or dilatation, and they are attributed to a variety of causes, frequently with a genetic basis [1]. Cardiomyopathies are commonly categorized into two groups: primary CMP which

IntechOpen

predominantly affects the heart and secondary cardiomyopathies which involve additional organ system complications. The primary CMP is subdivided in genetic, mixed, or acquired. The main genetic CMP is hypertrophic cardiomyopathy (HCM), arrhythmogenic CMP (ACM), left ventricular noncompaction, mitochondrial myopathies, etc. The acquired CMP is myocarditis, peripartum CMP, Taksubo, and tachycardia-induced CMP. Mixed CMP includes dilated and restrictive cardiomyopathies. Mechanical circulatory support (MCS) and heart transplantation (HT) serve as surgical interventions designed for cases of cardiomyopathies complicated by advanced heart failure (AHF). These procedures are typically pursued when sustainable medical or interventional treatments are not viable, and the affected individuals face a limited lifespan.

2. Mechanical circulatory support

Mechanical circulatory support (MCS) is used in the management of individuals experiencing advanced heart failure (AHF) or cardiogenic shock. These devices offer temporary hemodynamic assistance to patients facing severe heart failure with potential for recovery (bridge to recovery) as well as to those with irreversible heart failure where the goal is to extend the time available for transplant donor allocation (bridge to transplantation, BTT). Additionally, these devices may be utilized for providing permanent circulatory support to individuals who are not suitable candidates for HT (as destination therapy, DT) or as a bridge to decision. This final category encompasses patients who are hemodynamically unstable and require urgent MCS. However, the ultimate decision regarding MCS cannot be determined at the time of surgery [2].

2.1 Temporary mechanical circulatory support (TMCS)

TMCS may be employed for individuals experiencing acute heart failure or cardiogenic shock (CS). This includes extracorporeal membrane oxygenation (ECMO), extracorporeal life support (ECLS), and percutaneous cardiac support devices (**Table 1**) [3].

Criteria for CS are low cardiac index (<1.8 L/min/m2), systolic blood pressure < 90 mm Hg, and general signs of systemic hypoperfusion, such as elevated lactic acid in the absence of hypovolemia [4].

In a review article Atti [4] highlighted the stages of cardiogenic shock as per the Society of Cardiovascular Angiography and Interventions.

The objectives of MCS in CS include enhancing overall perfusion, optimizing coronary artery perfusion, and alleviating stress on the left ventricle.

Indications for mechanical circulatory support use are presented in **Table 2** [4].

2.2 Short-term MCS devices are intra-aortic balloon pump (IABP), Impella device, tandem-heart, and Veno-arterial ECMO

2.2.1 Intra-aortic balloon pump (IABP)

IABP is a left ventricle support device that augments the diastolic flow and secondary increases coronary perfusion by counter-pulsating balloon deployed in the descending aorta by femoral or axillary approach. The cardiac output (CO) is increased by 0.5 L/min, or after other data there is no improvement in CO [4].

DOI: http://dx.doi.org/10.5772/intechopen.1004875

Stages of shock	Haemodynamics	Biochemical markers	Description
Stage A at risk	Normotensive CI > _2.5 L/min/m^2 CVP < 10 PA sat > _65%	Normal renal function and lactate, elevated BNP	Patients not in Cardiogenic shock (CS) but at risk of developing CS (STEMI, or NSTEMI)
Stage B Beginning	SBP < 90 mm Hg, or MAP <60 or > 30 mm Hg drop from baseline Pulse >_100/min CI > _2.2 L/min/m2 PA sats >_ 65%	Normal renal function and lactate; elevated BNP	Clinical evidence of hypotension or tachycardia without hypoperfusion
Stage C Classic	SBP < 90; MAP <60 or > 30 mm Hg drop from baseline and drugs/device to maintain BP above these targets CI < 2.2 L/min/m2 PCWP>15 mm Hg RAP/PCWP >_0.8 CPO < _0.6 W/m2 PAPi<1.85	Lactate >_2 mmol/L: serum creatinine doubling or > 50% drop in GFR; elevated LFTs and BNP	Clinical evidence of hypoperfusion requiring medications/MCS beyond volume resuscitation to restore perfusion
Stage D deteriorating/ doom	Stage C + requiring multiple pressors or MCS devices to maintain perfusion	Stage C and deteriorating	Similar to stage C, but getting worse and failing to respond to initial interventions
Stage E	Hypotensive despite maximal support	pH < –7.2 Lactate >_5 mmol/L	Cardiac arrest (PEA or refractory VT/VF) with ongoing CPR or ECLS placement

SBP = systolic blood pressure, BNP=B-type natriuretic peptide, CI = cardiac index, CVP = central venous pressure, PA = pulmonary artery, MAP = mean arterial pressure, GFR = glomerular filtration rate, LFT = liver function test, MCS = mechanical circulatory support, BP = blood pressure, bpm = beats per minute, RAP = right atrial pressure, PCWP = pulmonary capillary wedge pressure, CHF = congestive heart failure, CPO = cardiac power output, PAPi = pulmonary artery pulsatility index, PEA = pulseless electrical activity, CPR = cardiopulmonary resuscitation, CS = cardiogenic shock; ECLS = extracorporeal life support, sat = saturation, VF = ventricular fibrillation, VT = ventricular tachycardia.

Table 1.
Stages of cardiogenic shock [3, 4].

Mechanical complications in acute myocardial infarction
Acute heart failure/acute or chronic heart failure
Post-cardiotomy shock
Acute cardiac allograft failure
Post-transplant RV failure
Refractory arrhythmias
Difficulty weaning from cardiopulmonary bypass
Prophylactic use for high-risk complex PCI
High-risk or complex ablation of VT
High-risk percutaneous interventions

Table 2.
Indications for mechanical circulatory support device use after [4].

It contains a double-lumen catheter and a pump console that controls the balloon. The triggers for balloon inflation are ECG or blood pressure. The balloon starts inflating at the end of aortic valve closure, or when diastole starts and rapidly deflating during the onset of systole increasing by this mechanism the coronary artery perfusion. This process involves generating a vacuum force that moves the blood into the aorta, thereby reducing the left ventricle afterload. With this mechanism of inflation-deflation, the coronary perfusion is increased, and LV afterload is decreased consecutively. The best outcome is attained when the balloon is correctly positioned into the aorta, and the inflation commences at the end of systole (correlates with T wave on ECG) and deflation starts at the end of diastole (R wave of ECG) [5]. Complications of IABP are vascular and nonvascular. Vascular complications are limb ischemia, arterial thrombosis, and retroperitoneal hematoma by abdominal aortic injury, which usually needs IABP removal and vascular repair of the artery. Arterial dissection, spinal cord ischemia, cholesterol embolization, and stroke, are less encountered. Balloon rupture with helium embolization is a rare complication and can cause ischemia or stroke [4].

2.2.2 Left ventricle to aorta support devices

Impella devices are widely utilized in contemporary medical practices, with approximately 40% of these being implanted in cases of cardiogenic shock [5]. These devices feature a rotary-flow axial pump, which comes in various capacities as 2.5, 3.5, 5.0 L, and most recently 5.5 liters. Notably, the 5.5 liter has a maximum flow of 6.2 liters, and this version eliminates the need for a pigtail catheter, thereby preventing potential issues like mitral valve entrapment [6]. The Impella devices are inserted either percutaneously or by surgical approach (impella 5.0 and 5.5) on femoral or axillary/subclavian arteries. The axillary approach provides the benefit of enabling patients to mobilize and walk. Each device consists of a pump motor and a flexible catheter, which is inserted into the aorta through the aortic valve [7]. An external console regulates the speed and flow, where increased speeds will lead to elevated blood circulation. The appropriate placement of the Impella device is monitored by radiography and echocardiography and by the pressure waveform generated by a sensor at the distal end of the pump. The pump may be positioned with the inlet in the ventricle and the output in the ascending aorta giving a pulsatile waveform because of the pressure differential between the two cavities. Complications arising from the insertion of the Impella device include hemolysis, aortic valve injury, arrhythmias, bleeding, vascular issues, such as leg or arm ischemia, and arterial bleeding or thrombosis. Apparently, Impella use has a higher risk of bleeding and vascular complications as IABP [7].

2.2.3 Left atrium to aorta support devices: tandemheart

The TandemHeart device is positioned between the left atrium and aorta consisting of a transeptal cannula terminating in the left atrium [5], which brings the blood to the iliofemoral arterial system. It comprises four components: the left atrial cannula (LA), a centrifugal pump, a femoral arterial line, and a control console [5]. The femoral cannula, with a diameter of 21 Fr, connects the femoral vein to the right atrium and traverses the septum into the left atrium. Blood from the left atrium is directed through the arterial cannula (15–19 Fr), entering the right common femoral artery. The extracorporeal centrifugal pump, equipped with a spinning impeller, propels the blood, generating a rotation speed between 3000 to 7500 RPM. The TandemHeart reduces PCWP and CVP and secondarily lowers LV and RV pressures, thereby diminishing the workload on the ventricles and oxygen demand. Contraindications of use include severe peripheral artery disease, left atrial thrombosis, and complications are related to insertion point (bleeding, arterial thrombosis, hematoma), limb ischemia, thromboembolism, or hemolysis [5].

2.2.4 Extracorporeal membrane oxygenation (ECMO)

ECMO is an adapted technique stemming from cardiopulmonary bypass and involves a blood pump, oxygenator, conduit tubing, and heat exchanger [4]. There are two types of ECMO, Veno-Arterial (VA) ECMO and Veno-Venous (VV) ECMO. The first aids the heart and lungs and the second supports primary the lungs. In VA-ECMO, the inflow cannula receives deoxygenated blood through a centrifugal pump in a membrane oxygenator and sent by an outflow cannula into an artery (VA) or venous (VV) system [8]. ECMO maintains cardiac output, is used in hypoxemic cardiogenic shock, and increases coronary blood flow. VA-ECMO increases LV afterload, LV end-diastolic pressure, and volume, and there is decreased coronary flow in diastole. That's the reason for adding another device as Impella or IABP to reduce afterload and preload [8]. Emergency indications for VA-ECMO are massive pulmonary embolism with right ventricular failure, sepsis-associated cardiomyopathy which ends with myocardial depression secondary to severe sepsis, and circulatory support in high-risk invasive procedures (TAVI, PCA, ventricular tachycardia) [9].

Complications of ECMO are vascular, neurological, hematological, and infections. Vascular issues in ECMO may manifest as limb ischemia linked to factors such as obesity, association with IABP, or arterial thrombosis, requiring surgical intervention [9]. Neurological complications are ischemic stroke and intracranial bleeding, coma, encephalopathy, and anoxic brain injury all with high mortality. Hematologic complications are bleeding which is the most common with 27 to 50% [4] due to low hemoglobin, anticoagulation, or acquired von Willebrand syndrome. Infections are very common and include cannula-site infections, or mediastinitis, pneumonia, sepsis [9]. A very common complication is thrombus on the circuit special in patients on ECMO for many days. Other complications are pulmonary edema, heparin-induced thrombocytopenia, air embolism, or acute kidney failure [4].

2.2.5 CentriMag and Rotaflow

CentriMag is a type of extracorporeal blood pump designed to assist or replace the heart function. Is completely magnetically levitated with no bearings with a very small prime volume of 31–32 ml. It can be used to assist one ventricle (RV or LV) or both ventricles [10]. The pump works by drawing blood from the patient body through a cannula, which is inserted into a large vein or artery. The blood is pumped through the centrifugal pump into the circulation. The system consists of centrifugal pump, console, and flow probe and can provide flows up to 10 L/min. An oxygenator can be attached to the tubing system for blood oxygenation. CentriMag pump offers comprehensive blood support, ensures effective decompression of both ventricles, enables potential patient mobilization, and can provide support for weeks or months. However, drawbacks include the requirement for surgical procedures during both implantation and removal. The device can be inserted by a median sternotomy or lateral thoracotomy [11]. Rotaflow pump is magnetically suspended on a sapphire bearing with no shafts. CentriMag pump has the best hemolytic performances

[12] comparatively with other centrifugal magnetically pumps as Rotaflow and Revolution. The outcome of using CentriMg device in Intermacs 1 critical cardiogenic shock is showing very good outcomes with 65% overall survivors after total explant [13].

2.3 Long-term mechanical circulatory support (LTMCS)

Long-term VAD can be categorized into intracorporeal, paracorporeal, and total artificial heart (TAH) types. In the intracorporeal category, devices as Heart Mate II, Heart Mate 3, EvaHeart 2, Jarvik 2000, and Heart Assist 5 are included. The paracorporeal group comprises devices like Excor Berlin Heart, while total artificial hearts include Syncardia TAH, first implanted in 1986 and the Carmat TAH, with its initial implantation occurring in 2013 [3]. We are introducing the Heart Mate 3 VAD as a prototype within the category of long-term VADs.

2.3.1 Indications for long-term VAD implantation

Durable mechanical circulatory support in the United States is primary utilized for two main purposes: serving as bridge to cardiac transplantation (BT) or as a permanent therapeutic solution for end-stage heart failure, commonly referred to as destination therapy (DT) [14]. The short-term mechanical circulatory support (MCS) group comprises MCS employed as a bridge to recovery and bridge to transplant, as well as long-term MCS for destination therapy (DT). Various clinical conditions, such as nonischemic cardiomyopathy, and myocarditis have the potential for reversing myocardial damage, making the weaning process from MCS feasible [14].

ISHLT Selection Guidelines for Durable left ventricular assist devices were detailed by Pagani [6] and are presented in **Table 3**.

Inclusion criteria
AHA Stage D Heart Failure
VO2 max <14 ml/kg/min, or > 50% predicted attainment of respiratory anaerobic threshold
NYHA functional class III/IV for at least 45 of the last 60 days, despite the use of maximally tolerated doses of drugs. The inability to tolerate neurohormonal antagonist medications (e.g., beta-adrenergic blockers) may lead to earlier consideration.
Exclusion criteria
Reversible cardiac dysfunction
Active uncontrolled coagulopathy
Inability to tolerate anticoagulation mandated for the LVAD
Renal disease that would significantly shorten life expectancy.
Hepatic disease that would shorten life expectancy
Lung disease that would negatively impact post implantation survival.
Diabetes, Severe peripheral vascular disease, moderate to severe aortic insufficiency, mechanical aortic valve that will not be converted to bio-prosthesis at the time of implantation, severe right ventricular dysfunction, severe cognitive impairment, advanced age with frailty, etc.

Table 3.
Inclusion and exclusion criteria for durable left ventricular assist device selection after [6].

2.3.2 Technique of implantation of heart mate 3 assist device

The conventional method for Heart Mate 3 left ventricular assist device (LVAD) implantation involves median sternotomy, utilizing the left ventricular apex for inflow cannula insertion and ascending aorta for outflow tract placement. This approach provides an improved view of the heart, but it comes with drawbacks, including increased risk of bleeding, potential right ventricular dysfunction due to full pericardial opening, and the likelihood of later adhesions if a second surgery for transplant is required. The procedure is done on cardiopulmonary bypass and beating heart but can be done off pump as minimally invasive procedure [15]. The inflow cannula is positioned at the left ventricle apex, 2 cm lateral from the left anterior descending coronary artery, and aligned parallel to the interventricular septum. The placement of the sewing ring is determined by placing a finger on the left ventricular wall, as identified by transesophageal echocardiography. Subsequently, the sewing ring is secured with interrupted Prolene sutures, and coring is performed while inspecting the ventricle for thrombi or residual muscular tissue, which may be removed.

The inflow cannula is then inserted into the left ventricle within the sewing ring and rotated to achieve the correct position at the outflow anastomotic site. An alternative cannulation site is the "Frazier point" on the inferior wall, situated laterally and posteriorly from the posterior descending coronary artery. The outflow graft is positioned parallel to the right ventricular margin within the pericardium, avoiding passage in front of the right ventricular outflow tract. The graft is then anastomosed to the ascending aorta using continuous Prolene sutures, with additional stitches applied for optimal hemostasis. In special circumstances, alternative courses for the outflow graft may be considered, such as through the transverse sinus or other arterial sites like the innominate artery descending aorta, supra-celiac artery, or axillary artery. The descending aorta is particularly utilized in lateral placement of the left ventricular assist device (LAVD) through lateral thoracotomy or in redo surgeries to avoid sternal reentry [15].

2.3.2.1 Complications of LVADS implantation

The main complications are bleeding, infection, thrombosis emboli, neurologic events, right heart failure, and aortic insufficiency. Bleeding is most common in the early postoperative period. Early bleeding is correlated with surgery, which is complex and with increased risk, and late is due especially to gastrointestinal bleeding (almost 60%) [16].

The occurrence of bleeding is influenced by various factors, such as antiplatelet and anticoagulation therapies, acquired Von Willebrand syndrome, and the angiogenesis cascade. Several treatment options, including arterial embolization, cauterization, and surgical procedures, are available to manage bleeding. Substances like somatostatin, omega-3 fatty acids, and digoxin are effective in reducing bleeding in patients with LVAD. Pump thrombosis, more common in Heart Ware and less in HM 3 devices due to reduced friction and shear stress, is addressed with antithrombotic therapies, antiplatelets, LVAD exchange, or urgent transplant. Neurological events, including hemorrhagic and ischemic strokes with an incidence of 5 to 30%, are associated with elevated blood pressure and anticoagulation. Right heart failure can occur early (within 30 days post-LAVD implant, proximately 5%) or late (after 30 days), requiring temporary right ventricular assist device implantation for early acute RHF or medical therapy for late RHF. Aortic insufficiency typically manifests in around 30% of cases within the first 2 years [17].

2.3.3 Outcomes

The results following implantation of **l**eft **v**entricular **a**ssist device (LVAD) generally show improvement, with a 1-year survival rate of 82.3% and a 2-year survival rate of 73.1% during 2015–2019 period in USA. However, it is crucial to note that adverse events remain significant, with infections (41%) and major bleeding (33%) being notable in the first-year post-implantation. In the Momentum 3 trial, the Heart Mate 3 LVAD did not demonstrate an enhancement in overall survival when compared to the Heart Mate 2. However, it did exhibit fewer instances of reoperation and bleeding complications, or aortic insufficiency [18].

3. Heart transplantation (HT)

Heart transplantation stands as the primary therapeutic approach for end-stage heart failure considered a gold standard treatment. The inaugural human heart transplant was conducted by Christiaan Barnard in Cape Town in 1967, marking the beginning of a procedure that has since been successfully performed worldwide [19].

3.1 Indications of heart transplantation

The ISHLT indications for HT are advanced heart failure, a VO2</=12 mL/Kg/min at maximal cardiopulmonary exercise test (or </=14 if the patient is intolerant to B blockers) or VO2 < 50% of the predicted. After the European Society of Cardiology HT is indicated in advanced HF refractory to medical/device therapy in absence of the contraindications [19].

3.2 Contraindications of HT

Contraindications of HT are absolute or relative. Absolute contraindications are age > 70 years old, Severe pulmonary hypertension (PAP > 50 mm Hg, PVR > 3 UI Wood irreversible with milrinone or levosimendan), Multisystem disease, severe lung disease, history of cancer, severe systemic infection, active smokers or drugs users, viral infection with severe organ damage. Relative contraindications are diabetes mellitus with organ damage or poorly controlled, irreversible renal dysfunction or liver dysfunction (cirrhosis), and severe obesity [19].

3.3 Donor selection

3.3.1 Donation after brain death (DBD)

In DBD donation organs are retrieved for transplantation from individuals who have been declared brain death. The evaluation of donors is initiated by confirmation of brain death and family agreed with donation the donor may be analyzed according to the guidelines [20]. The main parameters taken into account are age < 45 years, size, hemodynamic status and inotropic support, metabolism status, systolic function documented by echocardiography repeated daily, blood group and Anti-Human Leukocyte Antigen Compatibility, drug use or comorbidities as hypertension, dyslipidemia, or diabetes [19]. Coronary artery status is analyzed by the surgeon and or on angiography whenever possible.

3.3.2 Donors after circulatory death (DCD)

DCD donation can be performed in three ways: direct procurement followed by normothermic machine perfusion (DP-NMP) for storage and transportation, normothermic regional perfusion followed by procurement and storage in normothermic machine perfusion (NRP-NMP), and normothermic regional perfusion followed by procurement and static cold storage (NRP-SCS) [21]. Direct procurement with normothermic machine perfusion (DP-NMP) was initiated for the first time in Sydney in 2014, this approach involves pharmacological postconditioning of the organ. It includes the addition of erythropoietin and glyceryl trinitrate (GTN) to the preservation solution, combined with normothermic machine perfusion for transportation to the implanting hospital. Normothermic regional perfusion with normothermic machine perfusion (NRP-NMP) was developed in Papworth by Messer and after the circulatory death is confirmed extracorporeal membrane oxygenation is used to resuscitate the organs in situ but with the exclusion of the brain by clamping the cerebral arteries. After in situ heart revival, the cardiac function is assessed as in DBD donation, the heart is harvested in the usual way and placed on the normothermic machine perfusion device for transportation to the hospital. Normothermic regional perfusion-static cold storage (NRP-SCS) consists of ECMO perfusion after declaration of death and after heart function assessment, the heart is retrieved and preserved in cold storage if a short ischemic time is anticipated [21].

3.4 Heart assessment and retrieval technique on the donor

The contractility of the heart is judged by focusing on the right ventricle first then on the left ventricle. The whole heart needs to be inspected and the contractility assessed with very gentle maneuvers. The coronary arteries are inspected and palpated in all territories making sure they are free from coronary disease or malformations. During handling the heart attention is paid to the development of arrhythmias and drops in blood pressure. If the blood pressure, heart rate, and rhythm remain stable and in normal parameters, during the handling, this indicates a good-quality graft. Next, the pressures are measured directly in the right atrium, pulmonary artery, and left atrium. The filling of the heart is weighed to interpret these results correctly. The pressures must be in normal ranges to consider that the graft has a good function. All these information gathered during direct surgical assessment of the heart are analyzed together with the number of inotropes and vasopressors requirements, Echocardiogram, Electrocardiogram, and clinical history to reach a definite conclusion about using the heart for transplantation or not. All these data shall point towards a normal heart anatomically and functionally to accept the heart for transplantation. After the heart has been accepted for transplant the cardioplegia solution and preservation solutions are prepared. In our center, we use St Thomas cardioplegia to arrest the heart for explant and cold Ringer's for preservation during transfer to the implant center.

3.5 Donor heart explant surgery

Once the abdominal surgical team has completed the dissection of the organs that they are planning to retrieve. The full dissection of the heart including the great vessels is rendered. The SVC shall be dissected fully, including the azygos and right brachiocephalic vein. The aorta is dissected along the arch vessels. The IVC is also dissected circumferentially to warrant a clear view of the transection point of this vessel without risk of injury to the coronary sinus. Silk ties are passed under the innominate vein, left brachiocephalic vein, and azygos vein. Heparin is given at a dose of 300 IU/kg and waits for 3 minutes before cannulation. An antegrade cannula is placed in the ascending aorta, as high as possible. The interatrial groove of Waterston's Sonnengaard's is dissected to expose as much left atrial wall as possible in this area. For a correct explant first tie the silk ties placed under the veins structures mentioned above. This reduces the blood flowing into the heart. The next step depends on whether the lungs are being explanted for transplant or not. If the lungs are being used for transplant, we open the left atrial appendage, and a suction device is inserted to empty the left heart. If the lungs are not being used, then open the left atrium through the interatrial groove of Waterston or Sonnegaard's. Place a suction through this opening to empty the left heart. The following step is complete transection of IVC making sure not to injure the coronary sinus and preserve at least 5 mm of IVC with the heart. Once the heart is fully decompressed, apply the aorta cross-clamp as high as possible and start delivery of 1.2 liters of St Thomas cardioplegia. The heart shall arrest quickly and symmetrically, once the cardioplegia start to be delivered. This indicates good protection and patent coronary arteries. While administering cardioplegia there is forbidden to manipulate the heart. We may be sure that the heart is fully decompressed. Cold Ringer solution is applied on the heart surface but not ice to prevent thermal injury. After completion of the cardioplegia, the excision of the heart starts by dividing the right and left brachiocephalic veins. The SVC may be fully preserved with right brachiocephalic vein. The azygos vein is tied and divided below. The SVC is separated from the surrounding tissues until a clear view of the roof of left atrium is attained. Then the left atrium is cut close to pulmonary veins, if retrieving the lungs for transplant, it will be preserved 1 cm of tissue around the veins cuff. First, the cut goes to the roof of the left atrium until the level of aorta. Then, the IVC is completely divided preserving 5 mm at least and exposes the inferior pulmonary vein. Once this is achieved, the left atrial wall towards the IVC is cut. When doing this division, it may be to avoid inferior pulmonary vein damage and aim towards an inferior point located 1 cm from the lower margin of IVC to avoid penetrating the right atrium, which can happen sometimes. The above steps complete the excision of the right side of the heart. Now the remaining wall of the left atrium is divided, for achieving that we may lift gently the heart exposing the inferior and left lateral wall of the LA. Left atrium is divided by scissors preserving a small cuff of at least 1 cm attached to the pulmonary veins as well, for the use of lungs for transplant. The midpoint between left atrial appendage and the beginning of the left pulmonary veins is a good landmark to achieve this goal safely, the incision of the left side of the LA shall commence at this point. Once the inferior and lateral wall of the LA has been cut the only remaining attaching the left split is a few centimeters of atrial roof. This is accomplished very easily from the left side. Caution when dividing the LA always keep in mind to preserve no less than 2 cm of free wall around to facilitate the heart implant. The completion of the preceding steps means that the heart now is only attached to the mediastinum by the aorta and pulmonary artery. Proceed as follows, by dividing the ascending aorta at the level of the arch, to ensure to preserve all length. Consecutively aorta is separated from pulmonary artery until the bifurcation is clearly seen. If the lungs are being retrieved for transplant, then the PA is divided at the bifurcation level; differently, if the lungs are not being used, dividing the right and left PA branches will secure the PA whole length. Once the PA is divided, gentle traction to the heart up and downwards helps to divide the remaining tissue behind the aorta and PA to fully free the heart. The heart is then placed in cold Ringer's solution on a back table and inspected for injuries or eventual congenital anomalies. Double check for the great vessels integrity and quality. Cardioplegia 300 ml are administered at this point and packing the heart and transportation are the final steps of the process.

3.6 Heart preservation

To preserve the heart during transportation, we use cold Ringer's solution. These are other solutions used by different centers: University of Wisconsin (UW), Celsior and Histidine-Tryptofan-ketoglutarate (HTK). According to Yognan Li et al. [22], the University of Wisconsin solution shows improved survival results at 30 and 90 days. In our experience, Ringer's solution works very well. There are diverse means of transportation for the heart: the classical is 3 bags system, where the heart is placed in a plastic bag surrounded by the preservation solution and this bag is placed in another one with cold Ringer's, which is in turn placed in a third plastic bag with cold Ringer's too. Then it is placed in ice cooler. This method was tested and gave good outcomes. The recent innovation has been the introduction of the Sherpa pack Cardiac Transport system by Paragonix Technologies and Transmedics OCS (Organ Care System). In the case of the Sherpa pack, the heart is placed in a plastic container with the preservation solution; the container then is placed in a type of ice cooler. It has a probe that allows to know the temperature of the preservation solution around the heart. In the case of OCS Transmedics, the heart is placed in machine that perfuses the heart with oxygenated blood and a solution developed by Transmedics. This allows the heart to be transported on normothermic conditions and pumping. Both techniques are in progress and time will tell, which will add a definitive advantage.

3.7 Heart transplantation bicaval technique

3.7.1 Cardiectomy

The heart cannulation is done with the aortic cannula placed as high as possible in the ascending aorta, one metal tip venous cannula is placed as high as possible in SVC and another metal tip cannula in IVC. An antegrade vent cannula is placed in the ascending aorta for cardioplegia delivery and drainage. The patient is on cardiopulmonary bypass as soon as the new heart arrives at the transplant center. While cardioplegia is being given to arrest the heart of the recipient, the new heart is brought into the surgical field. The heart is inspected the LA appendage is sutured and 300 ml of cardioplegia are delivered. The recipient cardiectomy starts by transecting the SVC and dividing any remnant tissue by diathermy until the roof of LA is exposed. Then the aorta is transected and dissected free from the PA by diathermy taking care to injure the right and left PA branches. Then the PA is divided just above the pulmonary valve. When transecting these vessels, the length is very important for a comfortable anastomosis. On completion of these steps, proceeds the disconnect the heart from IVC. This maneuver involves cutting through the right atrium keeping a cuff of RA connected to IVC of about 2 cm. This will facilitate the IVC anastomosis during the graft implant. Finally, it is the turn to excise the heart preserving the LA only. Usually, the LA is very large in the recipient. If LA is small, the dissection of the interatrial groove is mandatory. The RA is opened fully and access the LA through it. The LA wall is cut just below the coronary sinus to make sure that we are preserving the whole LA.

3.7.2 Heart implant technique

The Prolene 3–0 extra long suture is used for left atrium anastomosis. Taking the new heart off cardiopulmonary bypass position the graft in the surgical field may be correct with LA appendage as a landmark on the left side. The anastomosis starts at the level of LA appendage with running sutures advancing towards the level of IVC. The bites shall include a good amount of tissue, the needle entry point about a minimum of 5 mm from the edge and no more than 3 mm apart to secure water tightness. After reaching the level of IVC, change direction and bring the other limb of the suture from the level of LA appendage and run towards the roof of the LA and tie. Now the next to anastomose is IVC and Prolene 4–0 is usually used. Here the cuff of RA that was preserved on the recipient IVC simplifies the anastomosis significantly. The wise advice is to anastomose the PA next with Prolene 4–0. The **rationale** for doing this anastomosis before the aorta is the fact that the wide surgical field allows a very comfortable PA anastomosis without having to push the aorta, which averts possible tear on the fresh aortic anastomosis line in the case that this was done first. It also grants a perfect view to adjust the length of the PA to prevent kinks and undue tension. Once the PA is done the aorta anastomosis is performed with Prolene 4–0. At this point, the heart is deaired and cross clamp removed. This is recorded as the time of graft reperfusion and end of the ischemic time. The target is to reperfusion the new heart in a time window of 4 hours from the moment of aorta cross clamp in the donor.

3.7.3 Taking the new heart off cardiopulmonary bypass

The rewarming phase of the new heart shall take at least 30 minutes. Then, very gradually start filling the heart and let it work harder bit by bit. Place atrial and ventricular pacing wires and pace at 110 or 110 beats per minute. Start inotropic support or vasodilators as required. And very slow wean from cardiopulmonary bypass. If distension of the heart occurs at any moment, stop the weaning process, go back to full cardiopulmonary bypass, wait another 15 or 20 minutes, and repeat the procedure. If there is left or right ventricular dysfunction, consider mechanical circulatory support starting with IABP first. In case of 3 attempts of unsuccessful weaning from CPB after correction of the electrolytes, column temperature, pH and optimizing inotropic support we can confirm the diagnosis of primary graft failure and place the patient on central Venous Arterial ECMO support. The patient is transferred to the ICU to wait for graft function recovery, which usually happens in the first 7 days post-transplant. The inotropic support reduction and echocardiography will inform about graft recovery to plan ECMO decannulation. Before closing the chest, hemostasis check is mandatory and to avoid pulling the heart and suture lines are very important because of the vulnerability of the heart.

3.8 Heart transplantation with bi-atrial anastomosis

Left atrial anastomosis is done as in the previous bicaval technique. The right atrial anastomosis is started at the superior part of atrial incision, and a continuous Prolene suture is carried inferiorly and superiorly to anastomose the septum and the lateral wall of the septum. The PA and aorta are sutured in the same manner as described on bicaval HT.

3.9 Heart transplantation with modified bicaval technique

The "modified" bicaval anastomosis involves performing left atrial anastomosis, inferior vena cava connection, and aortic anastomosis all while the aorta is clamped on cardiac arrest. Subsequently, the anastomoses of the superior vena cava and pulmonary artery are made on beating heart, after aortic clamp is removed. The method has the goal of shortening the warm ischemic time and secondarily to reduce the cardiopulmonary bypass time [23, 24].

4. Heart transplantation with LVAD explant

Performing heart transplantation in a patient with a prior LVAD implant is technically more challenging, necessitating the mandatory use of peripheral femoral cannulation and cardiopulmonary bypass to avoid catastrophic bleeding. Given that LVAD patients are typically on warfarin, it is common to administer vitamin K and fresh frozen plasma before surgery to reverse the anticoagulation effects. During LVAD implantation, the use of Gore-Tex membrane helps prevent adhesions between the sternum and the heart, facilitating easier explantation of the device [24].

4.1 Complications of HT

Complications following heart transplantation (HT) are associated with immunosuppressive therapy and can manifest either shortly after or long after surgery. Early complications encompass acute cardiac rejection, manifest as either cellular rejection or antibody-mediated rejection, primary graft dysfunction, cardiac tamponade, and right ventricular dysfunction. In some cases, temporary circulatory support may be required to facilitate heart recovery. Late complications include persistent graft rejection, coronary artery vasculopathy (CAV), and adverse effects of immunosuppressive medications, such as malignancy, chronic kidney disease, diabetes, hypertension, or infection. For early detection of acute rejection, frequent endomyocardial biopsies are essential, typically performed every week in the first month, or every second week for the second month, followed by intervals or every 3 months until the first-year post HT [25]. Long-term complications following HT include rejection, which can be present as heart failure or may even be asymptomatic, and coronary allograft vasculopathy (CAV). While coronary angiography has traditionally been the primary method for detecting CAV, the use of coronary computed tomography has been on the rise in recent times [25]. There is a significant risk of cancer in heart transplant patients, skin cancer being the most common [25]. Particular types of lymphoma or lymphoproliferative disease may also arise following HT. Additionally, other enduring complications include hypertension, diabetes, arrhythmias, and chronic kidney failure.

4.2 Outcomes after HT

The outcomes after HT depend on many factors as donor characteristics, donation process, type of donation (donation after cardiac death or donation after brain death), recipient history, indications for HT, surgical procedure, and postoperative early and late complications. Miklin et al. showed [26] in an analysis of the last three decades that there were no differences in HT survival between restrictive cardiomyopathy (RCM) and non-RCM but if are compared RCM, only radiation/chemotherapy patients are worse than all other RCM subtypes and notably amyloid RCM short-term survival has improved but long-term survival is still worse. Median survival post-transplantation increased from 8.6 years in decade 1982–1991 to 12.5 years in 2002–2009 [27]. Donor heart allocation system was revised in 2018 by the United Network for Organ Sharing. This new system has modified the approach of candidates on ECMO support have a shorter waiting list from 10 to 5 days and survival at 30 days has increased from 76.4 to 94.2% [26]. Recipient risk factors with worse survival were BMI > =30 kg/m^2, under-sizing the donor hearts <=20% does not affect survival but older patients had worse survival post-transplant. Recipients with idiopathic DCM had a better 1-year survival than ischemic cardiomyopathy. Donation after circulatory death has increased the donor pool by 48% [27] and the outcomes were similar to DBD donation. They had similar rates of rejection DCD group vs. DBD group 25 vs. 23% in the UK experience. Primary graft dysfunction (PGD) occurring in the first 24 hours after surgery rates are between 7.4 and 31% [26]. Recipients with PGD had a higher 30-day mortality 6.1 vs. 0.9% and lower 5 years survival compared with non PGD group [27]. Graft rejection can be cellular, or antibody-mediated and acute or chronic and cellular rejection (ACR) generally decreased *over* time. Cardiac allograft vasculopathy is the most important cause of death after 1 year from HT and represents a coronary occlusive disease of the heart due to inflammatory-immune mechanism, which affects predominantly the medium and distal part of coronary arteries. The proximal coronary artery lesions are related to donor-derived coronary artery disease. Surgical revascularization or PCI has both high mortality and is difficult. Other complications, which are limiting long-term survival, are malignancies especially skin cancer is the most common, with a rate of 1.7% at 1-year and 18.5% at 10-year survivors [27]. Renal failure is another long-term complication related to nephrotoxic effect of tacrolimus and despite recent improvements is worsening the 1-year survival [27]. Renal dialysis or kidney transplantation is necessary for long-term survival. Twenty-year survival following heart transplantation was presented by Hess et al. [28]. On more than 20,000 patients the greatest 10-year survival with no risk factors was 59.7% and 20-year survival was 26.2% [28].

4.3 Heterotransplantation and xenotransplantation

Heterotransplantation purpose is to provide therapeutic solutions for organ failure when human-to-human transplantation is not feasible because of the shortage of organs. The main challenges of heterotransplantation are immune rejection and the risk of transmitting infection from donor species to the recipient. Advances in immunosuppressive therapies, genetic engineering, and organ preservation techniques are being investigated to improve the success rates and safety of heterotransplantation procedures. Xenotransplantation, is a type of heterotransplantation when organs are transplanted from animals to humans, has a historical connection due to the perceived suitability of pigs as donors. Pigs are favored for their rapid growth, widespread availability, quick maturity, similar heart size to humans, low risk of infection transmission, and positive track record in genetic engineering. However, challenges arise from disparities in anatomy and physiology between pigs and humans, along with a significant divergence in the immune system relationship. The history of xenotransplanted hearts traces back to 1964 when James Hardy [28] performed the first attempt, transplanting a chimpanzee heart into a human who unfortunately succumbed within 90 minutes. Fast forward to 2022, when Dr. Bartley Griffith and his team [29] achieved a significant milestone by conducting the first successful pig heart transplant, which endured for 2 months. This groundbreaking procedure involved the use of a genetically modified heart, wherein 10 genes were either altered or knocked out. To enhance the compatibility and reduce the risk of complications like thrombosis, or complement activation, the researchers incorporated various human regulatory proteins [29]. Furthermore, a sophisticated immunosuppressive medication was added to prevent acute rejection and T-cell-mediated rejection. Despite these advancements, challenges persist, including religious barriers and potential risks, such as transmission of viral infections from pigs to humans [29]. While the likelihood of generating a new virus through mutations is low, it cannot be dismissed. Preserving solutions play a crucial role in enhancing survival rates by minimizing ischemic graft injury. In experimental studies, the preservation of pig hearts using oxygenated, 8-degree Celsius cold cardioplegia solution containing erythrocytes and hormones has significantly extended the preservation time [30]. In summary, xenotransplantation is a procedure that can offer a major reduction of the waiting list for heart transplants but there are still many questions and problems to be answered.

5. Conclusions

Mechanical circulatory support (MCS) and heart transplantation (HT) are complementary surgical interventions employed in cases of advanced heart failure. Despite existing guidelines and protocols, the decision to opt for MCS or HT is influenced by numerous factors. In the context of temporary mechanical circulatory support, the choice of devices is often determined by the expertise of the medical team, with VA-ECMO gaining popularity due to increasing use and improved outcomes. In the realm of long-term MCS, Heart Mate 3 has emerged as a dominant choice. Its popularity can be attributed to its smaller pump size, reduced thrombosis risk, and ease of implantation, even via thoracotomy. While heart transplantation is widely regarded as the optimal approach, its implementation is constrained by a limited pool of donors. Yet, progress in donations after circulatory death and encouraging strides in xenotransplantation hint at prospective solutions for surgical therapy, presenting a promising outlook for addressing the substantial rise in patients grappling with heart failure.

Author details

Alexandru Mihai Cornea[1*], Guillermo Rodriguez[1] and Alina Ligia Cornea[2]

1 Mater Misericordiae University Hospital, Dublin, Ireland

2 Beacon Hospital, Dublin, Ireland

*Address all correspondence to: cornea@protonmail.com

References

[1] Sinagra G, Merlo M, Pinamonti B, editors. Dilated cardiomyopathy from genetics to clinical management. (e-Book). Springer; 2019. DOI: 10.1007/978-3-030-13864-6

[2] Morgan JA, Civitello AB. In: Frazier OH, editor. Mechanical Circulatory Support for Advanced Heart Failure. A Texas Heart Institute /Baylor College of Medicine Approach. Springer; 2017. DOI: 10.1007/978-3-319-65364-8_7

[3] Voors AA, Ponokowski P, Bueno H, et al. 2016 ESC guidelines for the diagnosis and treatment of acute and chronic heart failure of the European Society of Cardiology. European Heart Journal. 2016;**37**:2129-2200. DOI: 10.1093/eurheart/ehw128

[4] Atti V, Narayanan MA, Patel B, Balla S, Siddique A, Lundgren S, et al. A comprehensive review of mechanical circulatory support devices. Heart International. 2022;**16**(1):37-48

[5] Brown DL, editor. Cardiac Intensive Care. 3d ed. Elsevier; 2018. pp. 478-493. ISBN: 978-0-323-52993-8

[6] Kirklin JK, Pagani F, Schueler S, Uriel N, Maltais S, et al. Mechanical Circulatory Support (ISHLT Monograph Series Book 14) Vol. 14, Ch 12. pp. 1-29

[7] Wong AS, Sin SWC. Short-term mechanical circulatory support (intra-aortic balloon pump, Impella, extracorporeal membrane oxygenation, TandemHeart): A review. Annals of Translational Medicine. 2020;**8**(13):829. DOI: 10.21037/atm-20-2171

[8] Chera HH, Nagar M, Chang NL, Mangual CM, Dous G, Marmur JD, et al. Overview of impella and mechanical devices in cardiogenic shock. Expert Review of Medical Devices. 2018, 2018;**15**(4):293-299. DOI: 10.1080/17434440.2018.1456334

[9] Pineton M, de Chambrun N, Brechot AC. Venoarterial extracorporeal oxygenation in cardiogenic shock: Indications, mode of operation and current evidence. Current Opinion in Critical Care. 2019;**25**(4):397-402. DOI: 10.1097/MCC.0000000000000627. hal-02285046

[10] Nagpal AD, Singal RK, Arora RC, Lamarche Y. Temporary mechanical circulatory support in critical cardiac care: A state of the art review and algorithm for device selection. Canadian Journal of Cardiology. 2017;**33**:110-118. DOI: 10.1016/j.cjca.2016.10.023

[11] Telukuntla KS, Estep AD. Acute mechanical circulatory support for cardiogenic shock. Methodist DeBakey Cardiovascular Journal. 2020;**16**(1):27-35

[12] Han D, Leibowitz JL, Wang S, He G, Griffith B, Wu ZJ. Computational fluid dynamics analysis and experimental hemolytic performace of three clinical centrifugal pumps: Revolution, rotaflow and centri mag. Medicine in Novel Technology and Devices. 2022;**15**:100153. DOI: 10.1016/j.medntd.2022.100153

[13] Mehta V, Venkateswaran RV. Outcome of centri mag extracorporeal mechanical circulatory support use in critical cardiogenic shock (Intermacs 1) patients. Indian Journal of Thoracic and Cardiovascular Surgery. 2020;**36**(Suppl 2):S265-S274. DOI: 10.1007/s12055-01060-6

[14] Saaed D, Feldman D, Banayosy AE, et al. The 2023 International Society

for Heart and Lung Transplantation guidelines for mechanical circulatory support: A 10-year update. Journal of Heart and Lung Transplantation. 2022;**42**(7):e1-e222. DOI: 10/1016/j.healun.2022.12.004

[15] Loforte A, Gliozzi G, Mariani C, Cavalli GG, Suarez SM, Pacini D. Ventricular assist devices implantation: Surgical assessment and technical strategies. Cardiovascular Diagnosis and Therapy. 2021;**1**:277-291. DOI: 10.21037/ctd-20-325

[16] Chaudry SP, DeVore AD, Vidula H, Nassif M, Mudy K, Birati EY, et al. Left ventricular assist devices: A primer for the general cardiologist. Journal of the American Heart Association. 2002;**11**:e027251

[17] Han JJ, Acker MA, Atluri P. Left ventricular assist devices synergistic model between technology and medicine. Circulation. 2018;**138**:2841-2851. DOI: 10.1161/circulationaha.035566

[18] Varshney AS, EM DF, Cowger JA, Netuka I, Pinney SP, Givertz MM. Trends and outcomes of left ventricular assist device therapy. JACC. 2022;**79**(11):1092-1105. DOI: 10.1016/j.jacc.2022.01.017

[19] Masarone D, Kittleson MM, Falco L, Martucci ML, Catapano D, Brescia B, et al. The ABC of heart transplantation-part 1: Indication, eligibility, donor selection and surgical technique. Journal of Clinical Medicine. 2023;**12**:5217. DOI: 10.3390/jcm12165217

[20] Copeland H, Knezevic I, Baran DA, Rao V, Pham M, Gustaffson F, et al. Donor heart selection: Evidence-based guidelines for providers. The Journal of Heart and Lung Transplantation. 2023;**42**:7-29. DOI: 10.1016/j.healun.2022.08.030

[21] Scheuer SE, Jansz PC, Macdonald PS. Heart transplantation following donation after circulatory death: Expanding the donor pool. The Journal of Heart and Lung Transplantation. 2021;**40**(9):883-888. DOI: 10/1016/j.healun.2021.03.011

[22] Li Y, Guo S, Liu G, Yuan Y, Wang W, Zheng Z, et al. Three preservation solutions for cold storage of heart allografts: A systematic review and meta-analysis. Artificial Organs. 2016;**40**(5):489-496. DOI: 10.1111/aor.12585, Epub 2015 Nov 2

[23] Ranjit J, Liao K. Orthotopic heart transplantation. Operative technique in Thoracic and Cardiovascular Surgery. 2010;**15**(2):138-146. DOI: 10.1053/joptechstcvs.2010.04.001

[24] Immohr MB, Boeken U, Bruno RR, Sugimura Y, Mehdiani A, Aubin H, et al. Optimizing anastomoses technique in orthotopic heart transplantation: Comparison of biatrial, bicaval and modified bicaval technique. Journal of Cardiovascular Development and Disease. 2022;**9**:404. DOI: 10.3390/jcdd9110404

[25] Arora S, Attawar S. Current status of cardiac transplantation I the 21st century. Indian Journal of Clinical Cardiology. 2022;**3**(2):94-102

[26] Miklin DJ, DePasquale C. Heart transplant outcomes in restrictive cardiomyopathy: UNOS registry analysis of the last three decades. JHLT Open. 2024;**3**:100031. DOI: 10.1016.j.jhlto.2023.100031

[27] Awad MA, Shah A, Griffith BP. Current status and outcomes in heart transplantation: A narrative review. Reviews in Cardiovascular Medicine. 2022;**23**(1):11. DOI: 10/31083/j.rcm2301011

[28] Hess NR, Seese L, Mathier MA, Keeblar ME, Hickey GW, McNamara DM, et al. Twenty-year survival following orthotopic transplantation in the United States. Journal of Cardiac Surgery. 2020;**36**:1-8. DOI: 10.1111/jcs.15234

[29] Wadiwala IJ, Garg P, Yazji JH, et al. Evolution of xenotransplantation as an alternative to shortage of donors in heart transplantation. Cureus; 2022;**14**(6):e26284. DOI: 10.7759/cureus.26284

[30] Steen S, Paskevicius A, Liao Q, Sjoberg T. Safe orthotopic transplantation harvested 24 hours after brain death and preserved for 24 hours. Scandinavian Cardiovascular Journal; 3 May 2016;**50**(3):193-200. DOI: 10.3109/14017431.2016.1154598